DEMENTIA
A Practical Guide

DEMENTIA
A Practical Guide

Marc E. Agronin, M.D.
Director of Mental Health Services
Miami Jewish Home & Hospital for the Aged;
Assistant Professor of Psychiatry
University of Miami School of Medicine
Miami, Florida

Practical Guides in Psychiatry
Daniel J. Carlat, M.D.
Series Editor

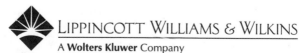

LIPPINCOTT WILLIAMS & WILKINS
A **Wolters Kluwer** Company
Philadelphia · Baltimore · New York · London
Buenos Aires · Hong Kong · Sydney · Tokyo

Acquisitions Editor: Charles W. Mitchell
Developmental Editor: Selina M. Bush and Lisa R. Kairis
Production Editor: Christiana Sahl
Manufacturing Manager: Benjamin Rivera
Cover Designer: Patricia Gast
Compositor: Lippincott Williams & Wilkins Desktop Division
Printer: R.R. Donnelley/Crawfordsville

©2004 by LIPPINCOTT WILLIAMS & WILKINS
530 Walnut Street
Philadelphia, PA 19106 USA
LWW.com

Printed in the USA

Library of Congress Cataloging-in-Publication Data
Agronin, Marc E.
    Dementia : a practical guide / Marc E. Agronin
    p. ; cm. — (Practical guides in psychiatry)
  Includes bibliographical references and index.
  ISBN 0-7817-3377-4
    1. Dementia—Handbooks, manuals, etc. 2. Dementia—Patients—Care—
  Handbooks, manuals, etc. 3. Caregivers—Handbooks, manuals, etc. 4.
  Geriatric psychiatry—Handbooks, manuals, etc. I. Title. II. Series
  [DNLM: 1. Dementia—diagnosis—Handbooks. 2. Dementia—
  psychology—Handbooks. 3. Dementia—therapy—Handbooks. 4.
  Caregivers—psychology—Handbooks. 5. Geriatric Psychiatry—methods—
  Handbooks. WM 34 A281d2004]
  RC521.A377 2004
  616.8'3—dc21   2003054512

Care has been taken to confirm the accuracy of the information presented
and to describe generally accepted practices. However, the author and publisher
are not responsible for errors or omissions or for any consequences from
application of the information in this book and make no warranty, expressed or
implied, with respect to the currency, completeness, or accuracy of the contents
of the publication. Application of this information in a particular situation
remains the professional responsibility of the practitioner.

The author and publisher have exerted every effort to ensure that drug
selection and dosage set forth in this text are in accordance with current
recommendations and practice at the time of publication. However, in view of
ongoing research, changes in government regulations, and the constant flow of
information relating to drug therapy and drug reactions, the reader is urged to
check the package insert for each drug for any change in indications and dosage
and for added warnings and precautions. This is particularly important when the
recommended agent is a new or infrequently employed drug.

Some drugs and medical devices presented in this publication have Food and
Drug Administration (FDA) clearance for limited use in restricted research
settings. It is the responsibility of the health care provider to ascertain the FDA
status of each drug or device planned for use in their clinical practice.

10 9 8 7 6 5 4 3 2 1

To the past . . .
The blessed memory of my grandparents,
Dr. Simon and Eva Cherkasky
and
Tany and Etta Agronin;

To the present . . .
The love and support of my wife Robin;

To the future . . .
My sons, Jacob, Max, and Samuel

Contents

Foreword

Physicians often ask, "Why should psychiatrists be interested in brain diseases such as the dementias?" In *Dementia: A Practical Guide*, Dr. Marc Agronin provides the answer. From the description of Alzheimer disease by psychiatrist Alois Alzheimer to the current methods of diagnosis and treatment, psychiatrists have much to contribute to the assessment and management of patients with this group of illnesses, as well as to those individuals providing day-to-day care. In a direct, readable fashion, Dr. Agronin nicely addresses many of the questions raised by patients, caregivers, and clinicians. He does not oversimplify things, and he does acknowledge that, at times, physicians cannot be as specific as they would like to be. This Practical Guide is just what the title suggests—useful, succinct, and accessible to the busy practitioner.

Peter V. Rabins, M.D., M.P.H.
Professor, Department of Psychiatry
Johns Hopkins School of Medicine, Baltimore, Maryland

Foreword

The information in this Practical Guide is aimed at a broad audience of clinicians, particularly students, residents, and fellows who see patients with dementia. It can also aid established physicians, especially those in primary care medicine and family practice (i.e., primary care physicians [PCPs]), whose patient populations include ever-increasing numbers of the elderly. This increase mirrors the significant growth of the elderly in general, particularly of individuals over the age of 85, that has been seen in the United States population. Most of these elderly patients with signs and symptoms of mental illness initially present to their PCPs rather than to psychiatrists, often describing vague symptoms like insomnia, pain, and headaches, so-called "tickets of admission" for this cohort of psychiatrist-avoiding individuals. This group includes those with cognitive dysfunction (often mild) that either is present alone or is comorbid with other problems, such as depressive or anxiety symptoms.

A recent survey found that PCPs feel reasonably confident in their abilities to diagnose and manage depression in their older patients. However, the same survey reported that almost one-half had not participated in any continuing medical education on or related to this topic during the previous 3 years. Furthermore, only about 40% of those surveyed referred even their moderately to severely depressed patients to a mental health specialist (1). This same situation undoubtedly occurs in elderly patients presenting with cognitive dysfunction, given that most elderly patients presenting to a PCP do not receive, no matter what the reason for their visit, a cognitive screening examination as part of their workup. This information underscores the need to provide relevant information to these first-line clinicians caring for elderly patients with cognitive and emotional symptoms.

Since 1991, the year of the first subspecialty board examination for added qualifications in geriatric psychiatry, only about 2,600 practitioners have been qualified in the United States. Because the body of knowledge in geriatric psychiatry is ever-expanding and unique, even those elderly patients referred to general psychiatrists may not be receiving optimal care. The availability of information regarding the rapidly expanding nosology of dementing illnesses to all practitioners is particularly important, not only because of the explosion in the numbers of elderly and the concomitant increase in the prevalence of dementia but also because of the clinical challenges inherent in the assessment of the cognitive and behavioral symptoms seen in these patients (2).

A truly useful and comprehensive Practical Guide for dementia must address the many complex issues still inherent to dementia care. It should base its approach on the current and evolving science in the areas of assessment, evaluation, diagnostic entities, and treatments for both the cognitive and behavioral aspects of the illness. Furthermore, sensitivity towards the education, and often the treatment, of family and caregivers must also be stressed. Finally, an effective guide should highlight and explain potentially useful research findings in key areas of dementia. This is particularly important because of the access to information, whether reliable or not, that the Internet gives to interested family members. The guide should therefore give clinicians the ability to look at the information found by the family and to separate the proverbial wheat from the chaff.

Dementia succeeds with all these facets, and thus, it should prove an important clinical resource for clinicians who treat the elderly. Dr. Agronin provides information about ongoing evaluation and empiric management that is based on current clinical guidelines and evidence-based outcome measures. The information is clearly organized for a better understanding of the pathophysiology of dementia and its associated clinical difficulties.

The following four comprehensive sections are highlighted in this practical guide: dementia assessment, its subtypes and their treatments, the associated psychiatric conditions, and the essential psychosocial issues. Vignettes of common clinical presentations are interspersed throughout the text. The Appendices contain pocket cards for key dementia areas that are important to both students and practitioners. This book is intended for use at the bedside; in the clinic; and particularly in the LTC setting, whether the individuals are in nursing homes or, increasingly, in apartments at assisted-living facilities. This book should become a frequent tool in these clinical settings for those caring for patients with dementia, as it provides specific and effective evaluation and management strategies for these long-term, corrosive disorders that cause such devastation for patients, families, caregivers, and society in general.

Caring for the elderly, particularly those with dementing illnesses, and their families is a privilege. Like all patients, they deserve the best that clinicians have to offer. *Dementia* is a useful, practical addition toward achieving that end in this clinical area, a sphere that is often challenging but that is always remarkably fulfilling and exciting as well.

Gabe J. Maletta, Ph.D., M.D.
Clinical Professor
Departments of Psychiatry and Family Practice and
Community Health
University of Minnesota, Minneapolis, Minnesota

REFERENCES

1. Harman J, Brown E, TenHave T, et al. Primary care physicians' attitudes toward diagnoses and treatment of late-life depression. *CNS Spectr* 2002;7:784–790.
2. Mulsant B. Geriatric psychiatry: challenges and opportunities. *CNS Spectr* 2002;7:780.

Preface

Do not cast me off in old age; when my strength fails, do not forsake me.

Psalms 71:9

The diagnosis of dementia or even the possibility of such a diagnosis is often greeted with fear and trepidation by those affected. The ensuing fears of losing one's mind and capabilities in the world and of being abandoned or 'put away' in an institution are contemplated as fates worse than death. The disease stealthfully encroaches in some individuals, robbing them of insight into their illness before they can truly appreciate what has happened. Others notice the changes building from week to week, month to month, and year to year yet resign themselves to the process. Still others fight the changes or those around them who insist that they cut back on the activities that once meant independence and integrity yet now carry the risk of disaster.

In its early stages, dementia is a disease that unifies patients, caregivers, and clinicians in a shaky alliance as patients try to cope with or to resist changes in cognition and function; caregivers attempt to minimize, ignore, or adapt to these changes; and clinicians seek to make a definitive diagnosis and to provide treatment for a disorder that can be elusive and that is usually incurable. The pitfalls in this alliance are clear—patients wrestle with fear and confusion that may sabotage their cooperation; caregivers struggle to overcome the overwhelming exhaustion, grief, and confusion they experience; clinicians must remain engaged despite a tendency to develop a fatalistic complacency.

Many of these factors are amplified as dementia progresses into the moderate and severe stages, ultimately culminating in a terminal state. Patients become robbed of those intellectual and functional abilities that made them unique individuals; caregivers can be overwhelmed with grief, guilt, and the drain of caregiving, a burden that, in turn, increases their own likelihood of dying by nearly 50%; clinicians must deal with the myriad problems associated with dementia, including delirium, apathy, depression, agitation, and psychosis, while still struggling to retain their ability to see and to respond to the humanity of each patient.

Those clinicians who read and use this book will find sufficient information teaching them about nearly every facet of dementia—its forms, pathways, pitfalls, and treatments. The book is designed to be a practical guide that can be brought into the clinic when one is evaluating and treating patients. I have endeavored to provide case vignettes and clinical tips to help the clinician move beyond a simple book knowledge of dementia and to hone his or her practical skills in assessment and treatment. I urge all clinicians, however, to integrate their own clinical styles into whatever techniques I suggest. Furthermore, they must understand that the rapid pace of research into dementia and its treatments may affect some of the information in this book, especially that relating to medication selection and dosing and Alzheimer disease.

With this in mind, the core theme underlying this book is *look for the human being behind the dementia*. In practical terms, a clinician who masters every facet of dementia may be knowledgeable but not necessarily wise or caring. Every individual with dementia is more than a diseased brain; he or she is also an ailing human who is surrounded by grieving caregivers with good hearts but limited amounts of time and patience. A busy and harried clinician can easily lose sight of these factors when he or she is working with demented individuals who can no longer express their own needs and wishes and who now are engaging in troubling behavioral problems.

Despite the efforts I have expended on this text, my sincerest hope is that the ongoing work of researchers and clinicians throughout the world will render this book obsolete by discovering definitive methods for the early diagnosis of and treatment for Alzheimer disease and other forms of dementia. In the interim, I hope that this work serves as an invaluable guide and resource for all clinicians wrestling with dementia in caring for their patients or in their own families.

Acknowledgments

First, I thank Dr. Daniel Carlat for giving me the opportunity to write this book on dementia for the Practical Guide in Psychiatry series. I also offer equally sincere gratitude to Charles Mitchell, my acquisition editor at Lippincott Williams & Wilkins, for all of his guidance, enthusiasm, and confidence; to developmental editors Selina Bush and Lisa Kairis; and to the production editor Christiana Sahl.

My wife Robin provided the warmest environment imaginable in which to write this book, as well as the love, support, and time to do so. My sons Jacob, Max, and Samuel have always provided necessary distractions from my labors; my sincere hope is that one day they will pick up a copy of their father's book on dementia and react quizzically to all the time and effort I spent writing about a disease that has been eradicated in their lifetimes. I also acknowledge the support of my parents, Ronald and Belle Agronin; my siblings, Robin and Greg Druckman and Michael and Ellen Agronin; and my in-laws, Fred and Marlene Lippman, who always provided a home away from home in which to work. I owe special thanks to Dr. Alan Cherkasky, whose practice of medicine has always inspired me and has provided me with practical tips on patient care.

Over the course of my professional training, I have been fortunate to work with many colleagues who, to this day, continue to lend an ear and to offer advice on many of the clinical topics in this book. They include Dr. Alan Bauer, Dr. Jimmy Levine, Drs. Steven and Randy Ugent, Drs. Stuart and Michelle Anfang, Dr. Gabe Maletta, Dr. Neal Foman, Dr. Elizabeth Crocco, Dr. Richard Polin, Dr. Stephen Scheinthal, Michael Druckman, Sean Sullivan, and Rabbi Eli Feldman. Dr. Maletta, a mentor and friend extraordinaire, graciously provided a foreword to this book. I also acknowledge my friends Jacobo Forma and Rabbi Heszel Klepfisz, two caregivers who embody the exemplary spirituality, wisdom, and devotion that is key to successful aging and coping. Many colleagues at the Miami Jewish Home & Hospital for the Aged (MJHHA) have provided advice and have served as models of care for the book: Dr. Robert Bergman; Judith Kessler, M.S., A.C.S.W.; Marilyn Goldaber, L.C.S.W.; Dr. Scott Crawford; Dr. Victoria Clevenger; Dr. Mairelys Martinez; Dr. Rita Gugel; Elena Selby, R.N.; Dr. Ricardo Blondet; Mindy Tucker; Beverly Beck, R.N.; and many other incredibly skilled members of the professional staff. I dedicate the chapter on working with caregivers to the memory of Rosemarie Terzo, an extraordinary nurse and administrator at the MJHHA. I particularly thank my friend and colleague Judith Kessler for her inspiration, support, and clinical expertise. My role at the MJHHA was made possible by the vision of Judge Irving Cypen and Hazel, his wife, who have devoted their lives to building the MJHHA into a world-class institution that has the ability to care for individuals with dementia in a comprehensive and compassionate manner.

I offer a special debt of gratitude to two individuals who were pivotal in the genesis of this work. Dr. Robert Bergman, Medical Director of the MJHHA, brought me into the wonderful institution that provided the essential inspiration and knowledge base for this book. He is a model clinician who embodies both the professional and ethical ideals to which this book is dedicated. Dr. Stephen Scheinthal, the closest of friends and my main consultant in dementia treatment, was a critical wellspring of advice and guidance for this book.

The most important inspiration for this book comes from memories of spending time seeing patients with my grandfather Dr. Simon Cherkasky, who practiced medicine in the small town of Kaukauna, Wisconsin, for over fifty years. He taught me many of the invaluable lessons that pervade this book—to work up each and every patient thoroughly, to treat them completely, and to make medical decisions based on clinical need rather than the availability of resources. This wisdom is crucial to the treatment of dementia. My grandmother Eva Cherkasky, his lifelong companion, provided from the warmth of her heart and her kitchen the true chicken soup for my soul. I hope that this book in a small way continues the educational and intellectual legacy of her own grandfather and my great-great grandfather, the beloved and well-respected teacher Rabbi Pesach Iser Gielczynski.

CLINICAL
ASSESSMENT OF
DEMENTIA

Dementia Defined

> **Essential Concepts**
> - Dementia refers to a spectrum of brain disorders, all of which involve cognitive impairment but vary widely in terms of the cause, course, and prognosis.
> - Dementia is more than just memory impairment; it involves impairment in multiple facets of cognition.

The term *dementia* has represented many different meanings and connotations over time. The word itself comes from Latin, literally meaning to be "without a mind." It is an ancient term that appears as both a disease state in Roman medical texts and a form of political sarcasm in the philosophical works of Cicero. In the past two centuries, the term dementia has most often been used to refer to brain disease characterized by intellectual impairment. The terms *presenile dementia* and *senile dementia* were frequently used to refer to disease states that developed before or after 65 years of age, respectively, and eventually the term *senility* became synonymous with dementia. In earlier diagnostic schemes, dementia had also been referred to as an organic mental syndrome and an organic brain syndrome. Regardless of the diagnostic term, dementia historically was viewed as a form of permanent brain damage.

DIAGNOSTIC CRITERIA AND ASSOCIATED FEATURES

According to the current diagnostic classification in the *Diagnostic and Statistical Manual of Mental Disorders*, Fourth Edition, Text Revision (DSM-IV-TR), *dementia* refers to the development of multiple cognitive or intellectual deficits that involve memory impairment of new or previously learned information and one or more of the following disturbances:

1. Aphasia, or language disturbance;
2. Apraxia, or impairment in carrying out skilled motor activities despite intact motor function;

3. Agnosia, or deficits in recognizing familiar persons or objects despite intact sensory function;
4. Executive dysfunction, or impairments in planning, initiating, organizing, and abstract reasoning.

These deficits result in significant impairment in both social and occupational functioning, and they represent a decline, often with an insidious onset and progressive course, from a previous level of functioning. Associated features of dementia that are not formally listed as part of the diagnostic criteria include personality changes, behavioral disruptions (e.g., agitation, disinhibition), apathy, depression, psychosis, anxiety, sleep disturbances, sexual dysfunction, neurologic symptoms (e.g., motor and gait disturbances, seizures), and delirium. Collectively, these symptoms result in a disorder devastating for both the affected individuals and their loved ones and caregivers. Therefore, the fact that the immediate caregivers of individuals with dementia have higher than expected rates of medical and psychiatric illness, especially depression, and increased mortality is not surprising.

CLINICAL VIGNETTE

Mr. Krone, a retired tailor, had immigrated to the United States from Poland at the age of 10 years and had spent most of his early life working in the garment industry in New York City. He later worked as a furrier, running his own business for more than 20 years. He was married for more than 60 years and had two grown daughters. Mr. Krone retired at the age of 70, and he and his wife moved to a retirement community in Florida. His wife passed away when he was 85, and, thereafter, Mr. Krone insisted on living by himself, despite his daughters' concern that his memory and physical strength had declined. Shortly after his 90th birthday, Mr. Krone fell and broke his hip. After the hip surgery, he was admitted to a long-term care facility for 2 months of rehabilitation, which eventually resulted in a permanent placement. Staff reported that Mr. Krone had significant cognitive impairment and symptoms of depression. He frequently spoke about his deceased wife, stating that he wished to join her. Six months after admission, Mr. Krone developed pneumonia, leading to his hospitalization. On his return to the facility, the staff noted that he was delirious, paranoid, and agitated. The delirium resolved after approximately 2 weeks, but Mr. Krone's dementia appeared to be much worse. He continued to be quite depressed and even overtly suicidal, with episodes of paranoia and agitation. These symptoms improved slowly after Mr. Krone was placed in a unit for residents with behavioral problems and was treated with psychotropic medications.

Many details of this case—a slow, insidious course; comorbid medical problems that lead to further decline; and associated problems, including depression, psychosis, agitation, and delirium—are typical for dementia, especially Alzheimer disease. As this case illustrates, long-term care placement is a frequent result.

EPIDEMIOLOGY

In the United States, approximately 4 million individuals have severe dementia, while another one to five million have mild to moderate dementia. The overall prevalence of dementia increases from between 5% and 7% at age 65 to 15% to 20% at age 75 and 25% to 50% after the age of 85. Some have predicted that, barring any major advance in prevention or cure, the number of older Americans who are most vulnerable to developing dementia (those 85 years of age and older) will nearly double in the next 30 years, causing a tremendous surge in the number of dementia cases. The estimated annual cost of treating dementia in the United States ranges from $40 to $100 billion, averaging nearly $200,000 per patient. Only heart disease and cancer incur greater economic costs.

CLASSIFICATION

Many different ways exist for classifying dementia subtypes, including classification by etiology, anatomic location, course, and prognosis. DSM-IV-TR lists the following major categories of dementia, without regard to a specific method of classification:

- Dementia of the Alzheimer type;
- Vascular dementia;
- Dementia due to one of the following: human immuno-deficiency virus disease, head trauma, Parkinson disease,

Huntington disease, Pick disease, or Creutzfeldt–Jakob disease;

- Dementia due to a general medical condition (specify the condition);
- Substance-induced persisting dementia;
- Dementia due to multiple etiologies;
- Dementia, not otherwise specified.

 KEY POINT

Of this list, Alzheimer disease is the most common, accounting for 50% to 70% of all dementias, while vascular dementia accounts for slightly more than 20%. Much overlap is encountered here because approximately 30% of patients with Alzheimer disease also have vascular dementia.

Dementia due to Lewy body disease is not listed in DSM-IV-TR, but it may account for nearly 20% of all dementias. All other types of dementia represent less than 10% of total cases, although considerable overlap is seen with Alzheimer disease and the other major types. Although the DSM-IV-TR describes the majority of dementias, it also obscures the great diversity of subtypes. This section reviews several approaches to classification and then presents a complete list of dementia subtypes (grouped by etiology) in Table 1.1.

Reversible Versus Irreversible

Between 10% and 30% of the presentations of dementia are potentially reversible when the underlying cause can be identified and treated. A more accurate description would identify several subtypes of dementia under this heading as arrestable and modifiable because treatment of the cause may only ameliorate the course of the disease without stopping the pathologic process. An example of an arrestable dementia is normal pressure hydrocephalus, in which treatment can reduce the hydrocephalus and can arrest the progression of dementia but cannot reverse the existing cognitive impairment. Alzheimer disease could be an example of a modifiable disease, in which treatment with specific medications may temporarily improve or stabilize cognition without altering the fundamental pathologic process. The major reversible causes of dementia are discussed in Chapter 11, and these include structural or

TABLE 1.1. Subtypes of Dementia, Grouped by Etiology

Etiology	Subtype
Primary cortical degeneration	Alzheimer disease
	Dementia with Lewy bodies (diffuse, mixed, cerebral)
	Frontotemporal dementia or Pick disease
	Primary progressive aphasia
Primary subcortical degeneration	Dementia with Lewy bodies (transitional and brainstem)
	Parkinson disease
	Corticobasal degeneration
	Progressive supranuclear palsy
	Multiple system atrophy
Cerebrovascular disease	Vascular dementia
	Large-vessel and small-vessel strokes
	Multiple lacunar infarcts
	Binswanger disease
	Cerebral autosomal dominant arteriopathy with subcortical infarcts and leukoencephalopathy (CADASIL)
	Cerebral amyloid angiopathy
Structural or traumatic injury	Neoplastic disease: brain tumors
	Paraneoplastic disease: limbic encephalitis
	Traumatic brain injury
	Dementia pugilistica
	Chronic subdural hematoma
	Normal pressure hydrocephalus
	Postanoxic state
	Post–coronary artery bypass grafting or postsurgical state
Toxic exposure	Substance-induced persisting dementia
	Medication-induced dementia
	Alcohol dementia
	Inhalant-induced dementia
	Wernicke–Korsakoff syndrome
	Toxic metal exposure (e.g., lead, mercury, manganese, arsenic)
	Wilson disease (copper poisoning)
	Toxic gas exposure (carbon monoxide, carbon disulfide)
Nutritional deficiency	Vitamin B_{12} deficiency
	Subacute combined degeneration
	Pernicious anemia
	Folate deficiency

TABLE 1.1. *Continued.*

Etiology	Subtype
	Niacin deficiency (pellagra)
	Thiamine deficiency (beri beri, Wernicke–Korsakoff syndrome)
Infectious disease	Bacterial
	Bacterial meningitis, encephalitis, or abscess
	Whipple disease (*Tropheryma whippelii*)
	Viral
	Viral meningitis or encephalitis
	Herpes simplex encephalitis
	Human immunodeficiency virus-1–associated dementia
	Progressive multifocal leukoencephalopathy
	Subacute sclerosing panencephalitis
	Encephalitis lethargica (sleeping sickness)
	Spirochetal
	Neurosyphilis
	Lyme disease
	Fungal
	Fungal meningitis, encephalitis, brain abscess
	Cryptococcal meningitis
	Parasitic diseases causing brain abscesses or cysts
	Prion diseases (transmissible spongiform encephalopathy)
	Creutzfeldt–Jakob disease
	Variant Creutzfeldt–Jakob disease
	Kuru
	Gerstmann–Sträussler–Scheinker syndrome
	Fatal familial insomnia
Organ failure	Uremic encephalopathy
	Hepatic encephalopathy
Endocrine disease	Diabetes mellitus
	Hypothyroidism
	Hyperparathyroidism (hypercalcemia)
	Cushing syndrome (hypercortisolemia)
	Addison disease (adrenocortical insufficiency)

TABLE 1.1. *Continued.*

Etiology	Subtype
Neurologic and metabolic disorders	Huntington disease
	Multiple sclerosis
	Marchiafava–Bignami disease
	Inherited storage diseases
	Adrenoleukodystrophy
	Metachromatic leukodystrophy
	Cerebrotendinous xanthomatosis
Inflammatory disease	Collagen vascular diseases
	Behçet syndrome
	Sjögren syndrome
	Systemic lupus erythematosus
	Vasculitides
	Granulomatous angiitis
	Lymphomatoid granulomatosis
	Polyarteritis nodosa
	Wegener granulomatosis

traumatic brain injury; the toxic effects of medications and other substances; vitamin deficiencies; infections; neurologic disorders; and neurologic sequelae of endocrine, metabolic, and inflammatory diseases.

Progressive Versus Nonprogressive

This distinction groups dementias based on their clinical course. Alzheimer disease is the prime example of a progressive dementia, whereas dementia due to traumatic brain injury is a nonprogressive dementia as long as no more trauma occurs. The goal of all current research is to develop treatments to make all forms of dementia nonprogressive and ultimately *curable* diseases. A related distinction based on pathologic course is *degenerative* versus *nondegenerative* dementia. Degenerative dementias are associated with either insidious pathologic processes that are not fully understood, such as those seen in Alzheimer disease or prion-associated disorders (e.g., Creutzfeldt–Jakob), or a specific progressive neurologic disorder, such as multiple sclerosis or Parkinson disease. Nondegenerative dementias result from episodes of brain injury, such as stroke or a traumatic injury, that are not necessarily recurrent events. However, this distinction can be subtle and subject to interpretation. For example, vascular dementia may appear to be an obvious form of nondegenerative dementia when it is clearly due to a single stroke. However, one could argue that the underlying atherosclerotic disease is actually a degenerative process.

Cortical Versus Subcortical

This distinction refers to the anatomic location of the dementia's pathology, identifying either the cerebral cortex or the cerebral subcortical regions, including the thalamus, basal ganglia, and brainstem regions. Basic differences between cortical and subcortical dementias are outlined in Table 1.2. Keep in mind that, although these clinical differences provide some guidance for diagnosis, they are not absolute. The most

TABLE 1.2. Cortical Versus Subcortical Dementias

Feature	*Cortical versus subcortical*
Memory	Memory impairment is present in both but more prominent in cortical dementia
Cognition	Aphasia, apraxia, and agnosia are cardinal features of cortical dementia, whereas slowed cognitive processing and disruptions in arousal and attention are more prominent in subcortical dementia
Motor behavior	Prominent psychomotor retardation is seen in subcortical dementia, especially early in course, associated with dysarthric speech, gait disturbances, and parkinsonism; less prominent changes are seen in motor behavior in cortical dementia until later stages
Motivation	Apathy is common to both but is perhaps more common in subcortical dementia
Mood	Depression is common to both but perhaps is more prominent with subcortical dementia
Pathology	Cortical dementia is associated with primary damage to the neocortex and hippocampus; subcortical dementia involves damage to the deep gray and white matter structures, including the thalamus, basal ganglia, brainstem nuclei, and frontal lobe projections

common cortical dementia is Alzheimer disease; however, it ultimately affects the subcortical regions as well. Similarly, subcortical dementias cause much of their cognitive impairment by damaging the neural white matter pathways to the cortex.

DIFFERENTIAL DIAGNOSIS

Having reviewed the basic classification and subtypes of dementia, the clinician must remember that not everything that looks like dementia is actually dementia. The differential diagnosis of dementia includes varying degrees of memory impairment that resemble, but do not equate to, early-stage dementia.

 KEY POINT

Many medical and psychiatric disorders either mimic dementia or exist comorbidly with it (delirium is a good example), making a quick determination of a clear diagnosis extremely difficult. To clarify the differential diagnosis, the most important information is always the level of memory and cognitive ability that predated any impairment. All comparisons begin there.

The flowchart in Fig. 1.1 presents an algorithm containing the various conditions and diagnoses that must be ruled out when dementia is suspected.

Age-Appropriate Versus Age-Inappropriate Cognitive Changes

The effects of normal aging on cognitive function and memory are quite modest, and they are often never brought to clinical attention. Nonetheless, the context of aging and the common fear of dementia among many older individuals sometimes lead to great concern over occasional memory lapses (sometimes whimsically referred to as "senior moments"). Such fears no doubt stem from the tendency seen throughout most of the past 100 years to equate aging with senility, suggesting that dementia was inevitable. The line between what is considered age-appropriate memory change

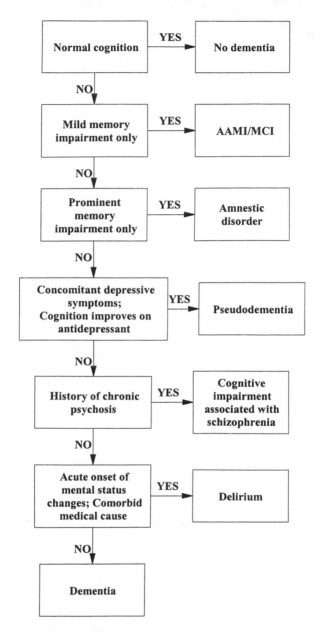

FIG. 1.1. Flowchart of differential diagnoses for dementia.
Abbreviations: AAMI, age-associated memory impairment;
MCI, mild cognitive impairment.

and age-inappropriate change is quite blurry, depending not only on subjective reports but also on diagnostic criteria that are still being debated.

A significant amount of research indicates that normal aging is associated with some deterioration in memory function. Deficits in attention and processing speed and accuracy can result in an overall decline in the short term (or immediate) memory. No uniform decline in memory occurs with aging, however. Although differences in performance generally favor younger subjects, these are small and they may be practically insignificant. In addition, factors such as environment (e.g., college versus retirement setting), testing familiarity, and expectations may affect test results, and many differences can be erased with training. Older subjects do perform better on some memory tests, an effect that may be attributed to increased overall knowledge.

Numerous terms have been used to describe memory loss that is greater than that which is seen with normal aging but less than that seen with true dementia. The two most widely used terms are age-associated memory impairment (AAMI) and mild cognitive impairment (MCI). These forms of mild impairment differ from the DSM-IV-TR diagnostic category of Cognitive Disorder, Not Otherwise Specified, in that the latter diagnosis indicates cognitive impairment that is presumed to stem from a comorbid general medical condition and that does not meet criteria for any other specific dementia. Neither AAMI nor MCI is believed to have a comorbid medical condition as an underlying cause.

The core diagnostic criteria for AAMI include an age of 50 years or older, subjective complaints of gradually developing memory failure that affects daily function, and a mean memory performance on neuropsychologic testing that is at least 1 standard deviation less than that seen in younger adults. Overall, the global intellectual function is otherwise intact, and neither a dementia diagnosis nor a condition known to produce cognitive impairment (e.g., stroke, brain trauma) is present. As many as 50% of older individuals may demonstrate AAMI. AAMI possibly represents a dementia prodrome because more than one-third of affected individuals later develops dementia.

The core diagnostic criteria for MCI differ slightly from those for AAMI, including subjective complaints of memory impairment by an affected individual or objective reports by a family member or physician, a mean memory performance on neuropsychologic testing that is at least 1.5 standard deviations less than the age-appropriate mean, and a score on the Clinical Dementia Rating Scale of 0.5. MCI does not involve impairment in activities of daily living or in global cognitive function. Like AAMI, MCI is associated with an increased risk for the later development of dementia. In one study, individuals with MCI had a 12% risk per year of developing dementia—primarily Alzheimer disease—compared with a 1% to 2% risk per year in individuals without MCI.

 TIP

If you have identified cognitive impairment in a patient but a specific dementia diagnosis is elusive, do not worry. The diagnosis usually emerges over time, but early intervention and decision making are important for all types of dementia. The tragedy is that this diagnostic uncertainty has made many clinicians complacent and willing to wait until they can be certain that a true dementia exists.

MORE DIFFERENTIAL DIAGNOSIS

When memory impairment is prominent but it is the only manifestation of cognitive impairment, a form of amnestic disorder may be the most appropriate diagnosis. Amnestic disorders are classified in DSM-IV-TR according to their cause (e.g., head trauma, general medical condition, substance induced, not otherwise specified), and they involve memory impairment for learning new information (anterograde) or recalling previously learned information (retrograde). When prominent symptoms of depression associated with cognitive impairment are present and when these symptoms improve with antidepressant therapy, the diagnosis of a pseudodementia ("fake" dementia), sometimes called a reversible dementia, would apply. The increased risk of developing a true dementia, given a history of pseudodementia, is discussed in Chapter 14.

Schizophrenia often presents with some degree of cognitive impairment that results from both the disorder itself and medication side effects. In older individuals with schizophrenia, more pronounced cognitive impairment may be related to the characteristic changes in brain structure, including cerebral atrophy and ventricular widening. Symptom overlap between schizophrenia and dementia can be confusing because both are associated with psychosis, apathy, and social withdrawal. However, older individuals with schizophrenia have a history of chronic psychosis and declining social and occupational function that began in younger adulthood.

Another key diagnosis that is critical to differentiate from dementia is delirium. The acute onset of mental status changes that characterize delirium should always prompt a thorough medical workup to establish an underlying etiology. Knowing a person's baseline cognitive status may help to distinguish dementia from delirium because dementia typically has a much longer and more insidious course. However, when such information is lacking, some clinical characteristics can be useful discriminators. These and other features of delirium are discussed in detail in Chapter 12.

2 The Dementia Interview

Essential Concepts
- The early diagnosis of dementia is challenging—the symptoms present insidiously, and patients, caregivers, and physicians often miss, ignore, or deny them.
- The early diagnosis of dementia is crucial for identifying and treating reversible causes, exacerbating factors, and associated psychiatric problems.
- The dementia interview should build a rapport with the patient and caregiver and should identify changes from baseline cognitive functioning.

In its early stages, dementia is not an obvious disorder. Every day, clinicians meet individuals in the community or see patients in clinical settings whom they would never guess have dementia. Casual conversation may not be revealing, and the friendly smile and graciousness of an older individual can easily cover up memory deficits, especially if a person's social skills are well preserved. In contrast, the stereotypical "demented" person is imagined to be extremely frail, aged, and either stuporous or agitated. Further distorting the image of dementia is the use of the term *demented* in everyday language to connote craziness, sickness, and even perversion. This limited view of dementia can lead clinicians to ignore important symptoms in someone who does not look the part and to assume that everyone who appears frail or disoriented is demented. The point of this chapter is to provide an understanding of the process of dementia and to inspire empathy for the millions afflicted with it.

Alarmingly, most individuals with early-stage dementia are not evaluated and treated at this time. Of the more than four million individuals in the United States with Alzheimer disease, fewer than half carry a diagnosis of Alzheimer disease, and fewer than half of that number are actually receiving any therapy. The often gradual and insidious course of dementia enables many afflicted individuals and their family members to ignore, deny, cover up, and/or compensate for early deficits.

Fear of Alzheimer disease and related dementias can reinforce the denial of illness despite the presence of obvious signs. Insight into early cognitive changes may be poor, hampering an individual's ability to recognize and then articulate the problem to loved ones. Compounding this problem is the failure of clinicians to diagnose dementia in anywhere from one-fourth to three-fourths of affected individuals, sometimes waiting years before referring them to geriatric specialists.

The evaluation often occurs in the setting of a crisis when a medical illness or a major life stressor (e.g., the death of a spouse, retirement) exposes the underlying cognitive impairment. Family members may express their alarm over the sudden change in their loved one's abilities. Frequently, this change is not sudden. More likely, the physical, psychologic, or social demands of a situation have overwhelmed the cognitively impaired individual's ability to hide his or her deficits. The increased family attention and scrutiny of an affected individual's behavior then reveal the deficits. The clinician must take all this into consideration when providing assessment, diagnosis, education, and some degree of family counseling.

CLINICAL VIGNETTE

Sonia was a 75-year-old woman with a lovely, affable demeanor. She was a retired teacher who had been widowed for 5 years. She had two daughters who both lived a plane ride away, and, for years, she had lived with her overprotective younger sister Rose in a retirement community. She was well loved by her internist, especially because, at each appointment, she and her sister would always bring a plate of freshly baked cookies to the office staff. Although, for several years, Sonia's daughters had noticed that she mixed up names and events when talking on the phone, Rose would always be on the line to correct her. Once, one of the daughters accompanied Sonia to a checkup with her physician, who reviewed her high blood pressure, arthritis symptoms, and wonderful chocolate chip cookies but did not raise any concerns about her memory. In response to the daughter's concerns, the doctor attributed any forgetfulness to "normal aging...," characterizing them as "...nothing out of the ordinary." Rose was suddenly hospitalized for congestive heart failure and died unexpectedly of complications. When Sonia's daughters arrived in town, they found that she was disheveled, grossly confused, and dehydrated. They took Sonia to her internist, anxiously wondering what was acutely wrong. A medical workup was unrevealing except for mild dehydration. Sonia now seemed completely unable to care for herself, and the daughters had to look for a suitable nursing facility. They could not understand what had gone wrong.

What is the moral of this case? A thorough evaluation of Sonia's mental status months or even years before Rose's death would have revealed significant cognitive deficits. Rose was a wonderful caregiver who had been able to keep Sonia well groomed, fed, and organized. As a younger sister, she did not want to believe that Sonia, her older, wiser, and more mature sister, was impaired. Sonia's gracious personality and appearance obscured any problems when she visited her busy physician. Without Rose, Sonia was incapable of organizing even the most basic daily activities, such as hygiene, appropriate dressing, and cooking. The stress of losing the presence and support of Rose, compounded with poor fluid and food intake, led to dehydration and delirium within days. Sonia's daughters were seeing the logical consequences of dementia in the absence of proper caregiving.

IMPORTANCE OF EARLY DIAGNOSIS

Early diagnosis is essential for the following reasons:

1. **To identify and treat reversible medical causes**, which sometimes lead to cognitive improvement.
2. **To make the correct diagnosis of dementia**, which can help to explain the presence of unusual, troublesome, and distressing behaviors, thus reassuring the concerned family members.
3. **To allow the individual to make critical life decisions** while he or she still retains maximal decision-making capacity, including financial and estate planning, advanced medical directives, and life plans. This capacity fades as the dementia progresses.
4. **To identify and treat associated psychiatric problems**, particularly depression, agitation, and psychosis, thus preventing excessive impairment, hospitalization, and early long-term care placement.
5. **To maximize safety** and to avoid catastrophe by setting limits on activities, such as driving; hunting; use of power

tools, firearms, or heavy machinery; and caring for young children.

6. **To provide treatment** to prevent or slow the progression or to ameliorate the symptoms of dementia, depending on its type.

 KEY POINT

Clinical trials comparing the use of cognition-enhancing medications with that of a placebo in individuals with Alzheimer disease have clearly demonstrated that those subjects on the placebo never attain the same level of improvement when they later are switched to active medication. Thus, the cognitive capacity lost by subjects without treatment is permanently gone. As with vascular dementia, brain damage from strokes can lead to permanent cognitive losses that could have been prevented or minimized by controlling important risk factors. Early diagnosis and treatment for each type of dementia can fundamentally shape its course.

WATCHING VERSUS REACTING

When the clinician notices potential signs or symptoms of dementia in a patient, what is the appropriate clinical threshold for reacting and pursuing a workup? Is simply watching the person for a while appropriate? Several suggestions to guide the approach follow.

1. In any adult younger than 65 (±5) years, the signs or symptoms of dementia more often reflect transient effects of medical illness or medications that warrant identification and treatment. Watching and waiting should never be an option. Signs and symptoms in children, adolescents, and young adults require immediate attention.

2. In adults 65 (±5) years of age and older, signs or symptoms of dementia may also reflect the transient effects of medical illness or medications, but they also increasingly reflect the presence of actual dementia, especially as patients enter their 80s and 90s. Watching and waiting for weeks to months may be appropriate only if screening tests and routine medical and laboratory examinations (see Chapters 3 to 5) are unrevealing. However, when screening tests suggest a problem, a full dementia workup should be pursued.

3. In the "old-old" (85 years or older), individuals, families, and clinicians often opt for more conservative approaches to working up the potential signs and symptoms of dementia. However, with more of the old-old living longer, healthier lives and the advent of symptomatic treatments for Alzheimer disease, the scope of dementia workups should never be arbitrarily limited. Although today, some may argue that doing a brain scan on a 100-year-old person is pointless, one should remember that, 30 years ago, the same argument was made about an 85-year-old person. Thus, age barriers are falling rapidly.

PHENOMENOLOGY OF DEMENTIA

The process of dementia can be viewed from the vantage points of both observers and patients. In many cases, the early symptoms are subtle and easily missed. In other cases, the symptoms are obvious to observers but unnoticed by the patient. The fear of dementia leads some individuals to over-react to normal memory lapses. Knowledge of how dementia presents is essential to clinical assessment; understanding what experiencing dementia is like can help clinicians to empathize with affected individuals and their caregivers and to provide optimal care.

How does dementia present? Several signs and symptoms that are listed in Table 2.1 may indicate the presence of early stages of dementia, particularly Alzheimer disease. The reader should, however, keep in mind the fact that these symptoms represent potential early signs and symptoms of dementia, not pathognomonic ones. Although all individuals with dementia present with one or more of these symptoms, many individuals without dementia may also demonstrate several of them. The key to making a diagnosis of dementia lies in identifying a pattern of symptoms and associated findings over time. Basic questions that can be used to identify these symptoms are found on Pocket Card A.1 in Appendix A.

What does a person with dementia experience? One way of thinking about Alzheimer disease is to picture a person's mind as a multilayered onion. Beginning in childhood, successive layers are added over the years as newly acquired memories and skills accumulate. Dementia is analogous to the slow peeling away of the onion, in which more recently acquired items are

TABLE 2.1. Possible Early Signs and Symptoms of Dementia

Sign	Symptoms
Forgetfulness	Commonly manifested as short-term memory loss for recently learned names, appointments, purpose of activities, points of conversation, and completed tasks or errands. An individual may repeat questions or requests. The degree of forgetfulness begins to interfere with daily activities and responsibilities.
Disorientation	Episodic confusion regarding the exact day, date, or location.
Impaired performance on daily tasks	Difficulty performing everyday tasks, such as preparing meals, running household appliances, cleaning, and hygiene (e.g., bathing, toileting, brushing teeth).
Impaired language	Increasing difficulty with selecting and using words. Sentences may become simpler or fragmented.
Impaired recognition	Diminished ability to remember or identify familiar faces, objects, sounds, and locations.
Impaired abstract thinking	Diminished ability to think clearly about issues, to discuss complex issues and to make logical connections between them, or to comprehend fully things that were previously understood.
Impaired judgment	Impairment in the ability to organize and plan and to make appropriate decisions or selections among several possibilities. A person may act in ways that were previously deemed uncharacteristic or inappropriate.
Changes in mood or behavior	Change in mood and behavior that may take many forms, including increased irritability, loss of emotional control (e.g., intense anger, frustration, tearfulness), abusive or inappropriate language, loss of pleasure in particular activities, and apathetic attitudes.

TABLE 2.1. *Continued.*

Changes in personality	The person may seem less sociable or more self-centered and may act out in disruptive or disinhibited ways. He or she may also seem more suspicious, fearful, or bothered by others, and reactions to everyday stress may be out of proportion.

lost first, followed by more remote memories and skills and eventually by even the most basic skills of eating, ambulating, and speaking. In its earliest stages, many individuals have only a vague sense that memory lapses and everyday forgetfulness are harbingers of dementia. The complaint of "I think I have Alzheimer disease" is more often interpreted as a sign of anxiety rather than as dementia, and it has no clear predictive value.

An individual's insight into his or her cognitive impairment varies widely as dementia begins; it is shaped by the demands of his or her mental activity and his or her overall level of self-consciousness, as well as the type of initial symptoms. For example, an accountant may notice subtle declines in mathematical ability more readily than does someone not engaged in number crunching. Changes in personality are usually not noticed by the affected person. The insight diminishes as the dementia progresses, and the affected individuals then become less likely to detect and understand their obvious cognitive impairment. Anxiety, depression, or agitation in an individual with advanced dementia is usually due to the immediate experience of confusion, discomfort, or disorganized thoughts rather than to the self realization that he or she is demented. Individuals in more advanced stages of Alzheimer disease commonly deny that they have any significant memory problems, and transient insights are quickly forgotten. First-hand accounts of the disease have given clinicians a view into this agonizingly slow process.

FIRST-HAND ACCOUNTS FROM CLINICAL INTERVIEWS

The first interview was conducted with an 85-year-old woman with vascular dementia and a mild to moderate degree of cognitive impairment. She does have some insight into her difficulties. In the interview, the patient's language is intact, but the vagueness of her descriptions should be noted. She is able to articulate the experience of searching an empty memory and the emotions that accompany it (I, interviewer; P, patient).

I: *Do you have a problem with your memory?*

P: *Oh, yes. Usually when I want to remember something, I have to dig down deep in my mind, in my memory. Sometimes I come up with something, sometimes not.*

I: *What is it like to have such difficulty with your memory?*

P: *Lonely...painful. Sometimes I accept what it is, sometimes I can't. I can remember back pieces of my life.*

I: *Where do you live now?*

P: *Isn't that funny, I don't remember. Isn't that horrible? I'm searching for it...I know I live someplace...where is my memory when I need it? All of it is very misplaced in my memory.*

The second interview is a record of a conversation with a 78-year-old woman with Alzheimer disease with moderate cognitive impairment and no insight into her dementia. Note that she attempts to answer every question but with some confabulation (responses not relevant to the question), mild language impairment, and frustration at being asked questions to which she cannot provide an answer.

I: *Do you have trouble with your memory?*

P: *No. None whatsoever. Not at all. I am. . .I don't have to forget anything. When you're with people like that, you sleep more...*

I: *Where do you live now?*

P: *With my husband, I think.*

I: *In what city do you live?*

P: *I don't know!* (angry tone of voice) *Because I'm telling you about my feet...in here* (pointing to her open mouth), *my teeth are so dry that for me to make a mistake is a problem. It's something that I have to take care of.*

I: *I would like to briefly test your memory. Could you please repeat the following three words: "apple, table, penny?"*

P: Well. Apple, tenna,...um,...you know,...this is not something I have to take care of because I'm leaving my husband too long...and he's sound asleep. No, not when I have this (pointing at me) to do. It is not something that I can't see him. I don't go for that.

I: Well, thank you for your time.

P: Oh, yes (smiling broadly), yes, thank you.

THE DEMENTIA INTERVIEW

The diagnostic interview for dementia has two main goals. The first is to establish a rapport with the patient and informant. Mutual and friendly cooperation lays the basis for a successful clinician–patient relationship from which all information and clinical responsibilities will flow. The second goal is to obtain all relevant history to determine the baseline level of functioning and to establish whether dementia is present. The baseline, defined as the most recent, sustained level of cognition and function, is perhaps the most critical component of the differential diagnosis.

Two challenges immediately present themselves. First, depending on the degree of cognitive impairment already present, the patient may not understand the nature of the interview, and/or he or she may react to it with confusion, suspicion, indignation, denial, or resistance. The individual may not even be competent to consent to the interview. A second challenge is that the informant, if present, may demonstrate some of the same attitudes as the patient. These two challenges limit the ability of the interviewer to accomplish the basic goals of establishing a rapport and obtaining needed history. Out of these challenges, however, come the following four principles for guiding the clinical interview:

1. **Interview to the patient's capacity.** As the interviewer begins to know the cognitive strengths and weaknesses of the patient, the type and manner of questions should be adjusted to match his or her ability to provide responses.
2. **Preserve the patient's dignity.** Always approach each patient, regardless of his or her known or assumed level of understanding, insight, or cognitive capacity, as if he or she is fully aware of the circumstances of the interview. The preservation of patient dignity is paramount in the ethical standards of clinical interviewing and in establish-

ing and preserving a rapport with the patient and caregiver. Doing otherwise can easily offend both.

3. **Obtain the patient's consent.** To the degree possible, the clinician should always seek permission from a patient to speak with him or her and should obtain consent to communicate with informants. One should avoid adopting an overly paternalistic attitude that can foster disregard for such permission. A breach of informed consent and confidentiality can be perceived by the patient as a slight, leading to negative impressions of the clinician, as well as noncompliance with the interview.

4. **Respect boundaries.** Respect the patient's and the informant's right to set time limits on the interview, to refuse to answer questions, and to limit access to informants. This respect ultimately results in the best possible chance to obtain necessary information.

These principles may seem obvious, but they actually require constant vigilance in a busy clinical practice. Their role in building a rapport and trust cannot be underestimated; guarding them carefully will enhance the principles of assessment and treatment discussed in this book. In particular, several essential components of patient dignity must be safeguarded, including the following:

- Respect for patient autonomy, decision-making capacity, privacy, and confidentiality;
- Opportunity for the patient to display strengths (e.g., ability to communicate in a native language) and to participate in life-affirming activities (e.g., religious observances) that are appropriate to his or her personal history and values;
- Freedom from embarrassment, humiliation, and inappropriate exposure;
- Provision (to the patient) of information regarding medical, social, and psychiatric factors appropriate to his or her personal values and level of understanding.

All these factors should be in place regardless of the patient's awareness of their presence or his or her awareness of situations that compromise such factors but that are apparent to outside observers.

CLINICAL VIGNETTE

Dr. W. was a geriatric psychiatrist in a busy clinic. When he interviewed Mr. Shapiro for a dementia assessment, he left the door to the room open and allowed an aide and a niece in the room without asking Mr. Shapiro for permission. The aide discussed several embarrassing behavioral outbursts by Mr. Shapiro in front of the niece and within earshot of another patient waiting in the hallway. Mr. Shapiro did not fully understand the nature of the interview, and, at several points, he cried out in Yiddish to Dr. W. *"der boich tute mir vey!"* ("My stomach hurts!"). Dr. W. assumed that Mr. Shapiro was merely acting out in a manner described by the niece, and, not knowing Yiddish, he merely smiled at him and ignored his cries.

Although Dr. W. was able to obtain adequate history about Mr. Shapiro, his undignified approach to this interview was inappropriate, and ultimately he missed the fact that Mr. Shapiro's behavioral outbursts were frequently caused by stomach pain and constipation. A stool softener, rather than the psychotropic medication that Dr. W. prescribed for him, would have been a better treatment for the agitation. Providing proper translation for Mr. Shapiro in a more relaxed and private setting would have allowed him as the patient to communicate something meaningful about his situation.

A wide variety of patients will present for dementia assessments, and the interview must account for all the special needs of these patients, including cognitive, sensory, and psychiatric impairments. Table 2.2 outlines the steps of a dementia interview for an older individual with potential cognitive impairment; it includes several handy tips for maximizing the factors just described.

TABLE 2.2. Guide to the Dementia Interview

---

1. *Preparation.* Before arrival, ensure that the patient is informed about the nature of the appointment, including the time, location, duration, types of questions, specialty of physician, and purpose. This process should be repeated at the time of the appointment to increase orientation, to maximize comfort and compliance, to ensure informed consent, and to minimize anxiety. Ask an informant to accompany the patient and request that he or she select an appointment time that works well for the patient's daily routine (e.g., avoid a time of day when the patient typically naps). Make sure that the interview setting is quiet, private, and free of distractions that may disorient or upset the patient and impair his or her ability to participate.

(continued on next page)

TABLE 2.2. *Continued.*

2. *Introduction.* Offer a formal introduction to the patient regardless of his or her potential cognitive limitations. This introduction should always include your name, title, specialty, and the purpose of the interview. Some patients may need more cues regarding the location and time of day, but be careful not to infantilize them or to overwhelm them with too much detail.

3. *Sensory check.* Always be aware of sensory impairment, especially hearing and visual loss. Do not assume that a nonverbal patient is aphasic—he or she just might not be able to hear you! When hearing impairment is a factor, always speak loudly into the better ear. Have an amplifying headset available for the patient. Use eye contact and gentle physical touches on a limb to maintain the patient's attention. Physical contact can also be useful for the visually impaired.

4. *Build rapport with patient and informant or caregiver.* Smile frequently and broadly. Maintain good eye contact, and, if appropriate, touch the patient in a reassuring manner. Use a soothing, yet audible, tone of voice. Inquire about their life history and family. Interview each patient as a person with a rich life, rather than as another individual with dementia. Speak to the informant or caregiver and inquire about his or her own experiences and stresses. Find areas of common interest to discuss. Listen to him or her in a relaxed manner, and make sure that, by the end of the interview, the informant knows how to get in touch with you if necessary. Solicit questions and answer all of them.

5. *Interview tips for more severely demented individuals.*
    Nonverbal behaviors may be the best (and only) information that the patient can provide.
    Use simply worded questions with a single idea (e.g., Do you feel sad? Are you afraid?).
    Questions may have to be "yes" or "no" rather than open ended.
    Do not rush questions. Be patient and wait for delayed responses.
    Provide language translation when necessary.

3 The Dementia Workup I:
History

Essential Concepts
The dementia workup. . .
- includes all components of standard medical and psychiatric history taking, with the addition of caregiver and home assessment;
- must incorporate a series of age-specific and dementia-specific inquiries to determine the risk factors for dementia and to identify individuals at risk of harm, abuse, or exploitation due to their cognitive impairment;
- addresses the mental and physical state of whole individuals, their environments, and lifestyles, *not* just the dementia.

That the author of the Sherlock Holmes mysteries, Sir Arthur Conan Doyle, was a physician should come as no surprise because the search for a medical diagnosis is a process not unlike the search for clues in a great mystery. Similarly, the dementia workup can be viewed as a medical mystery in which clues must be gathered about aspects of an individual's physiologic, psychologic, and social function to determine a diagnosis. The well-organized approach described in this chapter will help clinicians to identify quickly the key diagnostic factors in otherwise complicated geriatric cases.

The comprehensive dementia workup is described in its entirety in Chapters 3 through 5, and it includes the following components:

- The medical and psychiatric history and a review of symptoms;
- An assessment of the social environment and caregiver status;
- A physical and neurologic examination;
- A mental status examination with brief cognitive screening tests;
- Diagnostic medical tests: laboratory tests, brain scan, electroencephalography, and others;

- Neuropsychologic and functional testing.

The basic information needed for the dementia workup is listed on Pocket Cards A.1 through A.5 in Appendix A.

HISTORY

Components of the History

The first data gathered in any history are obviously the presenting problem and its history. Often, the clinician is unable to get a significant history from the dementia patient, so he or she has to rely on an informant and available medical records, which may themselves be limited.

CLINICAL VIGNETTE

Mr. Olsen was an 82-year-old World War II veteran and retired farmer who received his care at a Veterans Affairs hospital 100 miles from his rural home. He came to the dementia clinic with his wife after being referred by his primary care physician. During the interview, he stated that he was there to have his teeth examined. He denied having any significant memory problems, admitting only that "I'm a little forgetful at times." His wife described him as quite forgetful and noted that he did not sleep well. He sometimes wandered outside at night because he claimed to hear strange noises near the barn. She stated that he drives the car and still uses the electric carpentry equipment in his workshop. A note from his primary care physician described him as dependent on his wife to remember appointments and to manage his medications. A phone call to a daughter revealed a more extensive history of memory impairment, episodes of getting lost in the car, a car accident, a minor injury in his workshop, and episodes of agitation. Family members have had to go to Mr. Olsen's house several times in the middle of the night to calm him after his wife had spotted him circling the barn with a shotgun in his hand, yelling at an imaginary stranger.

Mr. Olsen is not atypical; in fact, his own attempts to present his history and the lack of crucial details from his wife illustrate why many individuals do not receive a diagnosis of dementia in a timely manner. A significant amount of time and energy may be required to track down informants who can present the most accurate account of the situation. When scheduling a dementia workup, the clinician should ensure that the best informant will be present, solicit the history ahead of time to anticipate gaps, and make referrals to dementia clinics whose staffs are well trained in gathering these data.

A description of the current behavior can range from subtle changes in daily functioning or personality to obvious and disruptive problems. The patient and informant should be asked to describe any current difficulties with memory or thinking, including how long they have lasted and whether they have progressed. If the responses lack focus, the interviewer should ask more specific questions about episodes of forgetfulness, disorientation, misplacing objects, getting lost in familiar settings, failure to recognize familiar people or objects (agnosia), difficulty performing everyday tasks (apraxia), word-finding problems (aphasia), and difficulty planning or organizing tasks (executive dysfunction).

The clinician should always determine whether any medical or psychiatric factors directly preceded the onset of symptoms or seemed to have worsened them. Several particularly relevant factors include a history of head injury, stroke, seizures, major depression, and the use of medications with known side effects on the central nervous system. Head injury and strokes can themselves cause dementia or can serve as risk factors and even triggers for Alzheimer disease (AD). Underlying vascular risk factors that should be identified include hypertension, high cholesterol, the use of tobacco and alcohol, peripheral vascular disease, atherosclerotic heart disease, and transient ischemic attacks. Seizures may suggest an underlying metabolic disorder or brain lesion. Major depression can sometimes lead to severe but reversible cognitive changes that are reflected in a pseudodementia, which, in turn, can increase the risk of dementia (see Chapter 14). Other important psychiatric symptoms include agitation, depression, psychosis, anxiety, apathy, personality changes, and any other behaviors that are unusual or uncharacteristic. The use of medications with strong anticholinergic, antihistaminic, and other side effects can impair cognition and can precipitate depression, psychosis, or delirium (Table 3.1 contains a complete list). In the history, obtaining a list of all prescription, over-the-counter, and herbal medications that are currently being taken is essential.

TABLE 3.1. Medication Side Effects that are Problematic in Dementia

Side effect	Manifestations
Anticholinergic	Memory impairment, confusion, delirium, dry mouth, blurred vision, urinary retention, constipation
Antihistamine	Sedation, dizziness, confusion, weight gain
Extrapyramidal	Stiff muscles, slowed gait, bradykinesia, tremor
Orthostasis	Blood pressure drop on standing, potential for syncope

⬥ KEY POINT

Anticholinergic effects may be the most worrisome medication side effects in the elderly because of their strong association with confusion and delirium. Anticholinergic effects oppose the actions of the neurotransmitter acetylcholine, which is critical to memory formation. Anticholinergic effects become especially deleterious when someone is taking an excessive dose of a single offending agent or several agents together, which then exert an additive effect. Commonly prescribed medications with anticholinergic properties are listed in Table 3.2.

TABLE 3.2. Medications with Anticholinergic Side Effects

Antipsychotics	Chlorpromazine (Thorazine), thioridazine (Mellaril), loxapine (Loxitane), clozapine (Clozaril)
Antispasmodics	Oxybutynin (Ditropan), tolterodine (Detrol)
Cardiac medications	Nifedipine (Adalat, Procardia), digitalis (Digoxin), isosorbide (Isordil, Imdur)
Diuretics	Triamterene (Dyrenium), hydrochlorothiazide, furosemide (Lasix)
H_2-blockers	Cimetidine (Tagamet), ranitidine (Zantac)
Tricyclic antidepressants	Amitriptyline (Elavil), imipramine (Tofranil), doxepin (Sinequan), clomipramine (Anafranil)
Others	Codeine, prednisolone, captopril (Capoten), dipyridamole (Persantine), warfarin (Coumadin), theophylline (Theo-Dur)

From Tune L, Carr S, Hoag E, Cooper T. Anticholinergic effects of drugs commonly prescribed for the elderly: potential means for assessing risk of delirium. *Am J Psychiatry* 1992;149:1393–1394, with permission.

Relevance of Social and Family History

The social history can establish a picture of premorbid social, occupational, and intellectual functioning that provides a context for change and enables comparisons with current deficits. For example, cognitive impairment relevant to mathematical skills (e.g., balancing a checkbook, paying for items at a store, performing calculations) will probably be more revealing in a college-educated individual who previously worked as an accountant. Similarly, apathy associated with dementia will be more revealing in a person who was always the life of the party or the perfect salesperson. A family history of dementia is rarely helpful in determining an exact diagnosis, but it may at least provide direction. For example, a history of cerebrovascular disease in first-degree relatives may suggest a higher likelihood of a vascular etiology for dementia. Family psychiatric history can be helpful in determining the individual's vulnerability to psychiatric symptoms, such as depression, anxiety, or mania.

REVIEW OF SYSTEMS

Each individual and informant should be questioned "from head to toe" to discern current symptoms and complaints that may be relevant to the patient's cognitive impairment. Reversible causes of dementia need to be identified, and the review of systems may offer clues to incipient problems that neither a routine medical history nor the physical examination is sufficient to identify.

 TIP

Attention to subtle neurologic complaints in the review of systems is particularly informative, including episodes of incontinence, weakness in a limb, disorientation, dizziness, or garbled speech. Such factors might point to unrecognized transient ischemic attacks or other cerebrovascular events that warrant more extensive workup. Chapter 8 focuses on vascular risk factors for dementia.

The review of systems should also obtain information about sleep, appetite, and psychologic stress. Major life events with the potential to induce strong adjustment reactions include retirement, financial loss, the death of a close family member or caregiver, relocation, family estrangement, and physical trauma. Individuals with dementia may overreact or react inappropriately to such major stresses and to minor events that frequently go unreported, such as a fender bender, a fight with a close friend, an embarrassing social indiscretion, or an episode of incontinence. Even individuals with memory impairment can become obsessively worried about a single event or a particular person. These reactions are important clues to the possibility of dementia.

ASSESSMENT OF ENVIRONMENT

Individuals with cognitive impairment can have an increased risk of self-injury, harming others, physical and mental abuse, neglect, and social and financial exploitation. Consider some situations that I have witnessed:

- A 79-year-old man with early AD signed over power of attorney to a daughter, who then promptly "borrowed" his remaining savings to finance her new house.
- An 84-year-old man with severe AD was living in a filthy, vermin-ridden apartment without nursing assistance because his mildly demented and paranoid wife was not capable of home maintenance and personal hygiene and was afraid that the social service workers were trying to persecute them.
- An 86-year-old man with mild dementia almost hit a woman pushing a baby stroller when his car careened through a parking lot and into a dumpster.
- A 75-year-old man with vascular dementia sustained broken ribs and multiple facial bruises after his daughter, who had a history of bipolar disorder and who had recently stopped taking her medications, flew into a rage and assaulted him after he was incontinent of urine on her couch.
- A 78-year-old wheelchair-bound man with moderate dementia living in a group home run by a kindly couple was confined to the inside most of the time due to the lack of wheelchair accessibility to the two-story house. The house lacked smoke detectors and fire safety equipment.

These troubling examples illustrate the need to gather information on both the care needs and the safety and adequacy of the social environment of the individual with potential dementia. The following questions can help:

- Does the home or other living environment provide adequate space, cleanliness, clothing, attention to hygiene, nutrition, and proper management of medications?
- Do bathrooms, stairs, kitchens, and other household locations account for the individual's physical limitations and sensory impairment?
- Does the individual receive adequate physical activity or therapy, sensory stimulation, and opportunities to engage in activities?
- Is the individual exposed to unsafe situations?
- Is the individual driving or using appliances or machinery against recommended advice?
- Does the individual need assistance taking medications?

The importance of these questions as part of the dementia workup should never be underestimated. The most brilliant workup and treatment plan becomes meaningless if the individual with dementia is returned to an unsafe environment. Chapter 15 contains information on educating caregivers on how to "dementia-proof " their home environment.

For individuals living in the community, their primary caregiver, commonly an elderly spouse or a daughter, is a vital part of assessment and treatment. If the caregiver is impaired, the individual with dementia can become excessively impaired. Moreover, the burden of caring for an individual with dementia, especially if he or she has associated behavioral problems, can increase the likelihood of depression, medical illness, and even the mortality of the caregiver. The dementia workup must therefore devote some attention to the physical and psychologic health of the caregiver.

CLINICAL VIGNETTE

Mrs. Sanders was a 67-year-old widowed woman with a history of breast cancer and depression. She served as primary caregiver for her 101-year-old mother, Deloris, who had AD. In addition to her poor memory, Deloris was frequently paranoid and agitated, and she would become verbally and at times physically abusive to her daughter. When her daughter refused to meet her outrageous demands, Deloris would sometimes smash her cane repeatedly against the front door and scream that she was being held hostage. Neighbors called the police to investigate on several occasions. Mrs. Sanders became increasingly helpless and depressed with the situation, but she agonized over the thought of sending her mother to a nursing home. She contemplated suicide and even ending her mother's life at the same time, but she always dismissed the thoughts, thinking that she did not "have the guts" to do it. She felt increasingly debilitated by chronic back pain and diarrhea, but medical evaluations were unrevealing.

Mrs. Sanders suffered from depression, fear, physical pain, social withdrawal, and even thoughts of both suicide and homicide, yet her situation as a caregiver is not unusual. Few clinicians who met Mrs. Sanders and her mother would have guessed the depth of her despair without careful, deliberate probing and consultation with other family informants. As Chapters 12 and 13 on assessing and treating agitation and psychosis explain, clinicians can do a great deal to improve such situations when they are aware of them.

Ideally, the caregiver has a sufficient degree of trust in and comfort with the clinician to portray his or her situation accurately. The following questions can elicit information from caregivers:

- What is your understanding of the affected person's disorder?
- How do you feel about the situation? Depressed? Hopeless? Helpless? Resigned?
- What is most burdensome about the situation?
- What social supports do you have? How helpful are they?
- Do you have help with specific caregiving jobs like hygiene, cleaning, and meal preparation? Is the help sufficient?
- Do you have time to yourself? If so, how do you spend it? Is it adequate?
- Do you have any current medical or psychiatric problems? If so, are you getting help?
- Have you been in touch with the local AD association or a support group?
- How do you see the future?

The answers to these questions will provide clinicians with a sense of how much the caregiver really understands the disease process and how it affects his or her own life. Sometimes just asking these questions and showing concern can be therapeutic for the caregiver. For more information on working with caregivers across settings, see Chapter 15.

The Dementia Workup II: Physical, Neurologic, and Mental Status Examinations

Essential Concepts

- The main goal of the physical and neurologic examination in the dementia workup is to identify any treatable medical factors that are causing or exacerbating the cognitive impairment.
- The mental status examination (MSE) provides a general screening for cognitive impairment and identifies psychiatric symptoms that may be causing or exacerbating cognitive impairment or behavioral problems.
- The Mini-Mental State Examination (MMSE) and the Clock Drawing Test (CDT) are popular and informative screening tools for dementia.

After the dementia workup has obtained all relevant history, the next logical step is to examine the patient's physical, neurologic, and psychologic functioning. The extent of each examination varies based upon the specialty of the clinician; for instance, a neurologist is likely to conduct a more thorough neurologic examination than other clinicians, whereas a geriatric psychiatrist's mental status examination may be longer and more specific than that conducted by a nonpsychiatrist. This chapter assumes, however, that all clinicians will conduct a thorough examination in each domain, then review records, and make appropriate referrals to fill in the gaps.

Sometimes, a complete dementia work-up requires the input from referrals to other clinical specialists in order to form the best diagnosis and treatment plan.

PHYSICAL AND NEUROLOGIC EXAMINATION

The main purpose of the physical and neurologic examination in the dementia workup is to identify potentially treatable medical factors that are causing or exacerbating the cognitive impairment. An outline of the basic examination is summarized on Pocket Card A.3 in Appendix A. From the moment an individual walks into the office for an evaluation, physical manifestations of medical illness may already be present. Neurologic signs and symptoms are commonly associated with particular types of dementia, and their presence can help to narrow the differential diagnosis (Table 4.1). One of the most important neurologic findings, especially in patients taking antipsychotic medications, is the presence of extrapyramidal symptoms.

TABLE 4.1. Neurologic Findings and Associated Dementia Types

Neurologic finding	Associated dementias
Extrapyramidal symptoms	Dementia with Lewy bodies, subcortical dementias (see Table 1.2)
Gait disturbances	Normal pressure hydrocephalus, vascular dementia, Parkinson disease, subcortical dementia, dementia with Lewy bodies, alcohol-induced dementia, tertiary syphilis
Hemiparesis	Vascular dementia due to large-vessel infarct
Frontal release signs	Frontal lobe dementia, other dementias in later stages
Myoclonus	HAD, Creutzfeldt–Jakob disease, uremic encephalopathy, late-stage Alzheimer disease
Peripheral neuropathy	Vitamin B_{12} deficiency, hypothyroidism, alcohol-induced dementia, heavy metal poisoning, uremic encephalopathy, HAD
Gaze paralysis	PSP
Pseudobulbar palsy	HAD, PSP, vascular dementia
Focal signs	Brain injury, vascular dementia, multiple sclerosis

Abbreviations: HAD, human immunodeficiency virus–associated dementia; PSP, progressive supranuclear palsy.

Manifestations of extrapyramidal symptoms include parkinsonism, dystonia, akathisia, and tardive dyskinesia. Parkinsonism refers to side effects that mimic symptoms of Parkinson disease and includes muscle rigidity, slowed movements (bradykinesia), and resting tremor. Muscle rigidity may manifest in a stiff or masked facial expression, in a shuffling or festinating gait, or in cogwheel rigidity.

 TIP

To test for cogwheel rigidity, place one hand on the patient's biceps muscle while grasping his or her hand and moving the forearm up and down. Feel for a ratcheting movement in the biceps muscle that feels as if the arm is moving on a cogwheel.

A parkinsonian tremor is rhythmic at three to six cycles per second and is most prominent at rest; it can be seen in the head, mouth, and limbs. Dystonia involves abnormal and painful contractions or cramps in a group of muscles and occurs less frequently. Akathisia involves an uncomfortable motor restlessness of the legs. Dyskinesia is abnormal, involuntary muscle movement that can affect any muscle group. Tardive dyskinesia is a syndrome that can occur spontaneously in late life or as a delayed (hence, *tardive*) reaction to antipsychotic medications. It tends to be more common in older women, and it may occur in 30% to 40% of older patients treated with conventional antipsychotics (e.g., haloperidol) during the first year of treatment, compared with fewer than 5% of patients treated with the newer atypical antipsychotics (see Chapter 13 for more information on these two classes of antipsychotics).

MENTAL STATUS EXAMINATION

The MSE is the heart of the dementia workup. As with the physical examination, the MSE begins the minute that the patient walks into the examination room, and it continues until the patient leaves. The basic components of a standard MSE include appearance, attitude and behavior, speech and language, affect and mood, thought processes, thought content, and cognition (see Pocket Card A.4 in Appendix A). The following sections highlight several unique aspects of the MSE during dementia assessment.

Appearance, Attitude, and Behavior

The very appearance of the patient (grooming and dress, gait, motoric activity, and facial expression) coupled with his or her attitude toward the interviewer and interview content provides clues to the current situation and the diagnosis. For instance, a patient who is unkempt or malodorous may require more assistance with dressing, grooming, bathing, or toileting. Lack of spontaneous motor movement may reflect apathy or parkinsonism, whereas motoric restlessness, such as wandering or pacing, may indicate agitation, agnosia (the patient does not recognize his or her surrounding and is exploring or attempting to leave), or akathisia. The facial expression may reflect underlying feelings of anxiety, depression, or agitation. Some individuals appear bewildered or impatient as part of their reaction to a sense of confusion or dislocation during an appointment. Other individuals may refuse to cooperate with the interview, or they may respond in a hostile manner, suggesting the presence of underlying fear or paranoia. The initial observations must be corroborated by further investigation.

Speech and Language

The characteristics of an individual's speech, including tone, volume, quality, and articulation, should be examined. In addition, the clinician should note the comprehension and expression of the patient's language, in which thoughts are transformed into language and language into thoughts. The clinician must ensure that the patient can hear the interviewer's questions so that he or she can respond. The most important form of language impairment in most forms of dementia is *aphasia*, which is characterized by underlying impairment in comprehension, expression, or both. Distinguishing aphasia from *dysarthria* and *aprosody* is important. Dysarthria is incoordination of the physical production of speech that is caused by muscle or nerve damage to vocal muscles or to relevant control centers in the central nervous system, especially the cerebellum. Lack of emotional tone characterizes aprosodic speech, which can result from stroke or head injury. Alterations or abnormalities in speech may also characterize some psychiatric conditions. For instance,

TABLE 4.2. Speech and Language Disturbances Seen in Dementia

Disturbance	Comprehension	Expression
Hearing loss	Intact; only for what is heard	Intact
Dysarthria	Intact	Incoordinated or garbled articulation, but language formation is intact
Aphasia (nonfluent/ Broca)	Intact	Impaired repetition; impaired grammar, telegraphic speech
Aphasia (fluent/ Wernicke)	Impaired	Impaired repetition; speech is fluent and melodic but not very intelligible due, in part, to multiple paraphasic errors (incorrect word choice or placement of word sounds)
Aphasia (conduction)	Intact	Impaired repetition; speech is fluent and intelligible but with paraphasic errors
Aphasia (global)	Impaired	Impaired, with some preservation of automatic speech

loud and pressured speech occurs in disinhibited and manic states. In some individuals, severe depression may render a voice almost inaudible. Impairment in generating names of items is called *anomia*. Descriptions of the major forms of language impairment are listed in Table 4.2.

Affect and Mood

Affect refers to the emotional tone of a patient that is observed by the examiner, whereas mood refers to the patient's subjective description of his or her emotion. Affect has also been described as the current emotional state, whereas mood is the more enduring or characteristic emotional state. Dementia may damage the brain's limbic system, an important component in the generation and shaping of emotions, or the frontal lobes, which help to determine the selection and appropriateness of emotional expression. In later stages of dementia, affect becomes a more accurate indicator of emotional state than does self-reported mood.

TIP

When you inquire about mood, a cooperative individual with more severe dementia may sometimes provide direct but inaccurate responses, such as answering "yes" or "no" to every question. If you simply ask "Are you sad?" to which the patient answers "yes," do not immediately conclude that an element of depression is present; you may find that he or she also answers "yes" when you ask if he or she is happy. When you suspect such a response style, ask multiple questions repetitively and then ask the opposite in a similar fashion. An individual who responds "yes" to every question or who does not respond consistently when asked these questions a second time is obviously not a reliable historian.

Common affective changes in dementia include increased irritability, lability (i.e., rapid fluctuations), and apathy. The clinical challenge is to determine whether fluctuations in affect constitute an actual mood disorder. Consider the following clinical vignettes.

CLINICAL VIGNETTE

Mrs. Wallach was an 81-year-old long-term care resident with a history of vascular dementia. During the day, she was noted to cry frequently without apparent reason. Sometimes she would begin sobbing after being startled by a loud noise. Nursing staff and family members expressed concern that she was severely depressed.

CLINICAL VIGNETTE

Mr. Klemt, an 88-year-old man with subcortical dementia, lived at home with his wife of 65 years. He sat impassively in his wheelchair all day, staring at the television and never initiating any conversation. He made very little movement in his chair. Although he was agreeable to suggestions made by his wife, he answered her perfunctorily with "yes" or "no" responses.

In each case, correlating the current affect and mood with other parts of the history and examination is important. For example, Mrs. Wallach had a history of frontal lobe and subcortical cerebral damage from strokes. She always denied feeling depressed, and she demonstrated good appetite and sleep. Her affect was more reflective of the neurologic syndrome *pseudobulbar palsy*, also known as *emotional incontinence*, than of depression or mania. Mr. Klemt, conversely, was more apathetic than depressed because he did not demonstrate any symptoms of depression other than his affect, and he put up no resistance to his wife's efforts to encourage more involvement in activities. Chapter 14 describes in more detail how to differentiate between dementia, depression, and apathy.

Thought Process

Disruptions in thought process may be symptomatic of the dementia itself or of an associated psychosis or another psychiatric disorder. Regardless of the causes, impaired thought processes can be seen when an individual attempts to answer questions and to provide history. Individuals with severe memory impairment may *confabulate*, providing responses either that approximate or that are not related to the question. They may overcompensate by providing a lot of extraneous or *circumstantial* information or marginally related or *tangential* information. When the frontal lobe circuits are damaged, an individual may *perseverate*—or present similar thoughts repeatedly—an occurrence that sometimes appears to reflect an obsession. As the patient's abstract thinking becomes more impaired, associations between ideas may become looser or less logical. Ultimately, demented thought processes can become quite *impoverished* and even *blocked* by the inability to equate words with ideas (due to aphasia) or to recognize the subjects of the discussion (due to agnosia). These changes may manifest as significant *response delay* or *latency* or even as *muteness*. The patient may, however, still be able to communicate even with severe aphasia, such as when he or she is expressing more automatic or overlearned forms of thought. The following clinical interviews illustrate disorders of thought processes due to dementia (I, interviewer; P, patient):

Mrs. Brill is a 69-year-old woman with a history of alcohol abuse, possible Alzheimer disease (AD), and severe short-term memory impairment suggestive of Wernicke–Korsakoff disease. Her dementia makes remembering and connecting thoughts nearly impossible for her.

> *I: Good morning, Mrs. Brill. How are you?*
>
> *P: Oh, yes, thank you, nice to see you. How are we?*
>
> *I: Fine, thank you. You are here to see the doctor.*
>
> *P: Yes (smiling), I thought you told me that...well, that is so nice!*
>
> *I: Do you know why you are here?*
>
> *P: Of course, for that thing I saw...can you believe it? She was there with us too.*
>
> *I: You are here to see the doctor.*
>
> *P: The doctor is here? OK, we had a lovely time there. That flower–set was right there, I think.*
>
> *I: Are you here to see Dr. Bell?*
>
> *P: Is that here for me, too? I guess I have to go now.*

Mr. Loren is a 92-year-old man with severe AD who demonstrates poverty of thought and response latency and who appears nearly mute except for several overlearned but aphasic responses.

> *I: Good morning Mr. Loren!*
>
> *P: Good morn–a, ah....*
>
> *I: How are you Mr. Loren?*
>
> *P: (30-second pause, while staring at examiner) Oh,... OK*
>
> *I: Mr. Loren, do you have any pain?*
>
> *P: (15-second pause) Ah...(silence)*
>
> *I: Do you have any pain, Mr. Loren?*
>
> *P: No.*

I: Thank you for seeing me today!

P: Thank...ank...yah.

Thought Content

In the assessment of thought content, several of the following factors are sought: delusions, hallucinations, and suicidal or homicidal thoughts. In addition, insight and judgment are evaluated. Delusions are false, fixed ideas, and, in dementia, they typically consist of paranoid, grandiose, or bizarre types. Some of the most common delusions include paranoid beliefs that a spouse is being unfaithful, that medications are poisonous, and that caregivers are trying to inflict harm. Hallucinations are false sensory perceptions that can be auditory, visual, and, less commonly, tactile and olfactory. Tactile hallucinations are suggestive of substance withdrawal, whereas olfactory hallucinations are associated with temporal lobe seizures. Visual hallucinations are sometimes associated with visual impairment, such as occurs in the rare Charles Bonnet syndrome in which an individual with no other psychiatric symptoms experiences vivid visual hallucinations (sometimes of small or Lilliputian people moving about) that typically cause little emotional distress. Visual hallucinations and delusions are common side effects of medications used to treat Parkinson disease, especially carbidopa (Sinemet). Auditory hallucinations are the most common type of hallucination encountered in psychotic states, including psychosis associated with severe depression.

In the MSE, distinguishing between confused thoughts and actual delusions or hallucinations is important, as the following example illustrates:

> Mrs. Ord was a 90-year-old woman with moderate AD. She told her doctor that her mother had come to visit her the other day. She began weeping, insisting that her mother told her that she was dying.

Was Mrs. Ord's experience a delusional belief that her mother had returned from the dead? Was it a delusion of misidentification, in which she believed that a visitor was actually her mother? Was she having hallucinations of seeing her mother? Was she merely confused by a recent visit by her daughter, who had always reminded her of her mother in looks and personality and who told her that she was not feeling well? All these are possibilities that should be explored in the MSE.

Treatment may hinge on the clinical distinctions between impaired thought processes and content due to dementia and those due to psychiatric illness. For example, a person with poverty of thought and speech latency may appear nearly mute and may be unable to communicate basic needs. When this is caused by advanced dementia, little can be done. However, when the cause is a severe, major depression, antidepressant medication could bring substantial improvement. Several of the following can aid in making these distinctions:

- **Onset.** Psychiatric impairment tends to have a more rapid onset, whereas impairment due to dementia is more gradual, except in the case of a large stroke.
- **Course.** Cognitive losses due to dementia tend to be permanent, whereas psychiatric symptoms may have a fluctuating course.
- **History.** Whether the individual experienced similar symptoms during previous episodes of psychiatric illness should be determined, as this indicates a higher likelihood of recurrent illness.
- **Associated symptoms.** Are other psychiatric symptoms that might provide clues present? For example, for the clinician who is wondering whether depression is a possibility, have changes in sleep, appetite, and energy that support a diagnosis of depression occurred?
- **Consistency.** Are the impairments in the patient's thought process consistent with the stage of dementia? For instance, severe poverty of thought in an individual with early-stage dementia would not be consistent with the cognitive changes during this stage; severe depression may therefore be a more likely explanation.
- **Response to treatment.** Impaired thought processes due to dementia will not respond to psychiatric medications, whereas targeted psychiatric symptoms may respond.

Suicidal and Homicidal Thoughts

The clinician must inquire about suicidal and homicidal thoughts because individuals at high risk of dementia are also at high risk of committing suicide. In the United States, older white men with medical problems, chronic pain, and significant psychosocial losses represent the group at highest risk of completed suicide. This risk can increase during the early stages of dementia when an individual may be reacting to increased cognitive impairment, especially if associated depression and/or impairment in judgment is present. Caregivers especially may be at risk of suicidal and even homicidal thoughts or behaviors directed toward an ailing spouse or parent. Although suicide-homicides in the elderly are rare, these are typically seen in a couple in which one spouse is quite ill and the other spouse (usually the husband) is overwhelmed by the burden of caregiving.

Passive suicidal thoughts are a more common form of suicidal ideation that are seen in dementia, taking many forms. An individual may express a sense of hopelessness or disgust over living and a lack of concern or even a wish that they either would not wake up in the morning, would die soon, or would be killed in some manner. On the borderline between passive and active suicidal ideation lie indirect life-threatening behaviors, which consist of unsafe behaviors that can potentially lead to injury or death, such as a refusal to eat, to take medications, or to receive medical treatment.

Feelings of hopelessness, depression, or anger may drive active suicidal ideation, but an intact executive function is required for the suicidal ideation to pose a risk of being carried out. Consequently, such ideation will become more vague and less organized as dementia progresses. Some individuals in early stages of dementia will confide their thoughts to family or clinicians, whereas others will make preparations without signaling their intentions to anyone. In later stages of dementia, individuals begin to lose the capacity to organize and carry out a plan; however, in rare cases, they may be assisted by family members.

MSE questions that can probe for suicidal and homicidal ideation include the following:

- Do you sometimes feel that life is not worth living?
- Do you ever think that it would not matter if you did not wake up in the morning?
- Are you tired of living?
- Have you ever had thoughts about hurting yourself or someone else?
- Have you had thoughts of suicide?
- Have you ever thought of ending the life of your loved one? Of killing them?

Although the last two questions are certainly the most direct and must eventually be asked, the first series of questions can sometimes provide a gentler lead-in to engage the patient and to encourage discussion. If someone responds "yes" to any of these questions, follow-up questions must determine whether the individual has a plan (e.g., overdose), the means to carry out the plan (e.g., a stash of pills), and the intent to do so (e.g., "if I don't recover, I would end my life"). Knowing whether the individual has ever attempted suicide in the past and whether a family history of suicide exists is also critical.

For an individual who lives either alone or with a caregiver in the community, the risk of suicide must be investigated, and appropriate preventive measures must be taken aggressively. In long-term care, many individuals are often too incapacitated to carry out a stated plan (e.g., a wheelchair-bound, deconditioned individual threatening to jump out a window), but they should not be underestimated. The follow-up questions should explore the full range of thoughts and emotions with respect to the suicidal or homicidal thoughts to determine the relative risk of something happening and also to uncover the feelings of sadness, hopelessness, helplessness, worthlessness, confusion, and desperation that are being communicated.

 KEY POINT

Whenever suicidal thoughts are reported, a clinician should search for the presence of other symptoms of depression. Even seemingly innocuous comments or transient feelings of hopelessness can indicate an untreated depressive disorder. By taking such expressions seriously, clinicians can send an important message of empathy and concern to the patient and family, which itself may be life-saving.

Insight and Judgment

Insight depends on the following factors: memory function, intelligence, abstract thinking, and self-consciousness. These factors determine the extent to which individuals can remember insights from one day to the next, their understanding of the disease process and their ability to recognize a change in their condition, and the degree to which they are aware of their own changing self. All these cognitive abilities begin to deteriorate in progressive dementia, so that any degree of insight that is present early on in the disease process will eventually disappear. In the MSE, the assessment of insight determines an individual's awareness of their cognitive impairment, and it can be gauged through several simple questions as follows:

- Are you having any memory problems?
- Do you have trouble thinking?
- Have you noticed anything wrong with your mind?

The degree of insight that an individual retains during the early stages of dementia can be a double-edged sword. Good insight into memory impairment can lead some individuals to be more cautious and to accept assistance; conversely, this insight can lead to anxiety, depression, and even panic in other individuals who react to their growing sense of confusion and difficulties in maintaining independence. Poor insight can hamper an individual's level of cooperation with treatment. He or she may resist efforts by caregivers to help, despite the fact that his or her attempts to drive, to care for other individuals, to use machinery or appliances, and to manage finances can be highly unsafe, unwise, or potentially disastrous. At the same time, poor insight may spare an individual the horrifying realization that he or she is losing his or her mind.

 TIP

When you are assessing an individual who appears to be in total denial of possible dementia, do not rush to confront him or her or any caregivers with a diagnosis. Focus on reaching points of agreement with respect to his or her needs; after all, this person is being seen in a clinical setting for some reason. Use points of agreement as a springboard to further assessment and treatment.

CLINICAL VIGNETTE

Mr. Lee was a 78-year-old retired electrician who presented to a memory disorders clinic with his wife for an appointment arranged by his primary care physician. Mr. Lee thought he was there to see a foot doctor, and he became angry when told otherwise. Mrs. Lee was unsure what the problem with her husband was. Despite a MMSE score of 18 of 30, which indicated a moderate degree of cognitive impairment, Mr. Lee only acknowledged that his memory was failing "like anyone else at my age!" Both Mr. and Mrs. Lee did agree, however, that they needed to move to a setting with more assistance. Instead of informing the Lees of the likelihood that Mr. Lee had dementia, the physician offered to have them meet with a social worker to discuss housing options; they readily agreed. During the course of the meeting, the social worker suggested that Mr. Lee have a more thorough assessment in the clinic to facilitate finding an appropriate facility. Thus, Mr. Lee went for neuropsychologic testing, which indicated a strong possibility of AD. At the same time, Mr. Lee's primary care physician, whom Mr. Lee had known and trusted for many years, ran all of the relevant dementia screening tests. When all test results were available, the physician and the social worker at the memory disorders clinic then met with Mr. and Mrs. Lee and suggested a possible diagnosis of AD. The diagnosis was couched in the context of providing medication to improve memory and an offer to assist with the transition to an assisted-living facility. Mr. and Mrs. Lee were more accepting of the diagnosis and of the offer for assistance because they had come to trust the staff at the clinic and had been given time to absorb the test results.

In the case of Mr. and Mrs. Lee, or similar individuals, the clinician should never hide or "candy coat" a diagnosis. The duty of a clinician is to provide honest and accurate results and clinical impressions. However, the appropriate time, situation, and manner in which to present this information should be considered. One should not rush to communicate clinical impressions until all relevant data has been gathered, even when a diagnosis is obvious.

It is important and sometimes difficult to respect a family's guidelines on what to tell the affected individual since it may want to shield the patient from the diagnosis. Clinicians' instincts are to present medical findings and diagnostic impressions honestly to the patient. With the elderly with dementia, this information often has to be presented in a simple manner that is free of diagnostic terms that may not be understood or that may prompt unwanted anxiety in the patient. When a person's medical decision-making capacity is compromised, the closest family members must fill in. They may not want to tell their loved one the exact diagnosis. Although the clinician may disagree with a family's judgment and may try to provide another perspective, ultimately he or she must respect the family's decision if he or she agrees to remain the patient's physician.

Judgment describes an individual's ability to make appropriate decisions. It depends not only on an individual's abstract abilities but also on his or her ability to discriminate between safe and unsafe and right and wrong and to maintain an awareness of social etiquette. Impaired judgment can range from minor lapses to humiliating indiscretions to even dangerous miscalculations. Consider the examples presented below:

CLINICAL VIGNETTE

Mr. Carp was a 68-year-old man with early AD. He was still driving despite his daughter's warnings to stop. One day he was pulled over by the police for failing to stop behind a school bus with its lights flashing and the stop sign displayed. When confronted by the police officer, he appeared incredulous when he was informed that driving around the bus was illegal.

CLINICAL VIGNETTE

Mrs. Green was a 78-year-old woman with vascular dementia who lived alone in an apartment. One evening, she came running out of her smoke-filled apartment screaming that there was a fire. Several neighbors rushed in to discover that she had turned on her oven with a cardboard box of food inside. When she was asked why she had done it, she seemed oblivious to the danger.

In both vignettes, an individual made a poor judgment that led to unfortunate consequences. These lapses in judgment reflect both a loss of knowledge of particular rules and a lapse in social etiquette. The best way to assess judgment in individuals with dementia is to ask family and staff about such incidents, rather than relying on specific screening questions.

Cognitive Screening

The goal of the cognitive screen is to qualify and to quantify the presence of cognitive impairment that may already be suspected by the results of the workup thus far. The ideal dementia screening instrument is quick, simple to use, and reliable, independent of examiner training and patient age, education, and cultural factors, and it has excellent sensitivity and specificity for dementia. Of course, such a test does not exist. However, several standardized instruments are available for use, and all focus to varying degrees on some of the following domains: attention, concentration, orientation, language skills, motor ability (praxis), word and object recognition, and visuospatial ability. If the examiner finds that a high index of suspicion for dementia exists after a screening, the individual should be considered for more comprehensive neuropsychologic testing and perhaps more extensive workup (detailed in Chapter 5). The most widely used cognitive screens are the MMSE and the CDT.

The administration of both the MMSE and CDT takes 10 to 20 minutes, and the information learned from each is complementary. When time is more limited, a condensed form of both, the Mini-Cog, can be substituted.

Mini-Mental State Examination

The MMSE is a 30-point scale assessing orientation, memory registration and recall, attention, calculation, language, and constructional ability. First published in 1975, the MMSE (and its variants) has remained the most popular screening instrument for dementia. This is probably because it is relatively simple and quick to administer, taking anywhere from 5 to 10 minutes, and because it provides a relatively high degree of both sensitivity and specificity for dementia. It also has established norms based on age and level of education. The disadvantages of the MMSE include its limited scope for frontal lobe and right hemispheric impairment and the fact that differences in administration and scoring can lead to inconsistent results.

ADMINISTRATION OF THE MINI-MENTAL STATE EXAMINATION
The patient is asked the questions and told to do the following tasks in order as listed on the test, without prompting or help from anyone else present in the room. The final score is based on a total of 30 points. However, if the patient has severe visual impairment, he or she may not be able to read or write a sentence or copy the intersecting pentagons. In that case, those items should be skipped, and the results are scored from a total of 27 points. For a visually impaired person, the person administering the test also has to adapt the task of naming objects, as described later. Administering the

MMSE to an individual who has severe hearing loss is difficult, if not impossible; one should consider having some amplified headphones on hand for these cases. For individuals who do not speak English, some clinical sites have translated the MMSE into other languages to meet the communication needs of their clients. If a translated version is in use, the clinician should keep in mind that a standardized format is no longer being used and that, as a result, no established norms are available for determining the best cutoff point for making clinical decisions about dementia. Another challenge to using a translated version is selecting an appropriate substitute for the word "world" to spell backward, as well as a substitute for the expression "no ifs, ands, or buts."

The key to administering the MMSE is maintaining a consistent method of asking questions and scoring because nuances of both can lead to score alterations in both positive and negative directions. The instructions described below for each question are based both on the published MMSE and on the author's own experience across a variety of clinical settings, including several dementia clinics. Individual technique may differ in small ways, but it should be used consistently and in concert with that of colleagues.

Orientation.   Ask the patient to tell you the (a) year, (b) season, (c) date, (d) day, and (e) month. Score 1 point for each correct response for a possible score of 0 to 5. Some clinicians allow a point for the date if it is only a day off. Ask the patient to tell you the current (a) state, (b) county or country, (c) town or city, (d) building or location (e.g., hospital, clinic), and (e) floor. Score 1 point for each correct answer for a score of 0 to 5. For the patient to say "hospital" even if he or she does not specify the full name is acceptable.

Registration.   Tell the patient that you wish to test his or her memory. Name three objects slowly and clearly, and tell the patient to repeat them back to you. Examples include "apple, penny, table" or "ball, flag, tree"; make sure that the objects are unrelated in terms of category and that they do not rhyme or alliterate excessively (e.g., you would not want to say "ball, fall, mall" or "bat, boy, blue"). After you have named all three, determine a score for the patient from 0 to 3 based on the patient's initial repetition. Repeat the word list, and allow several trials for the patient to repeat all three words successively.

Attention and Calculation. Ask the patient to start with 100 and subtract 7 from each number. Stop after 5 subtractions (93, 86, 79, 72, 65). Score the patient from 0 to 5 based on each correct subtraction. For example, if the patient responds with "93, 90, 83, 80, 73," he or she would receive 3 points, while "99, 98, 97, 90, 89" would receive 1 point. If the patient refuses to perform serial 7s or he or she cannot even attempt it (perhaps due to low education), you can substitute the task by asking him or her to spell the word WORLD backward (some examiners ask to spell it forward first). Make sure that the patient hears you clearly articulate the word WORLD instead of WORD. Score 1 point for each letter in the correct order, for a score from 0 to 5. For example, DLORW would receive 3 points, DLW would receive 3 points, and LDORW would receive 1 point. The spelling task is not an automatic substitute for serial 7s, so do not put it in just because you fear the patient cannot perform them.

Recall. Ask the patient to recall the names of the three objects learned earlier. Score 1 point for each recall for a score from 0 to 3. Some examiners (and caregivers in the room) are tempted to prompt the patient ("it's a type of fruit"), but this is not allowed. Do not score any prompted responses; however, you may want to assist his or her recall after the fact for your own assessment of the severity of his or her short-term memory.

Language and Praxis
Naming. Show the patient a watch and a pencil (or pen) and ask him or her to name the objects, scoring 1 point (total score of 0 to 2) for each correct response. This task may help to reveal both agnosia and expressive aphasia. If someone cannot see the objects due to visual impairment, you can either skip this item and score the total out of 25 (you will also have to leave out reading, writing, and pentagons) or place the objects in his or her hands, asking to identify them (although this technically assesses for a different type of cog- · nitive skill than visual naming).
Repetition. Ask the patient to repeat "no ifs, ands, or buts" after you. Be sure to articulate the phrase clearly and loudly. Score 1 point for an exact repetition. The most common mistake is for an individual to drop an "s" ("no if, and, or buts"), in which case they do not receive a point. This item can be extremely difficult for a hearing-impaired individual or for someone for whom English is not his or her first language as

the expression may not be familiar. With such individuals, be sure to say the sentence extra slowly and loudly. Allow only one trial on this item.

Three-Stage Command. Hand the patient a piece of blank paper and ask him or her to "(a) take the paper with your right hand, (b) fold it in half, and (c) put it on the floor." Score 1 point (possible score of 0 to 3) for each correct action. Several variations include asking the patient to fold the paper in half once for the sake of clarity; asking the patient to place it in his or her lap if he or she is in a wheelchair or has limited mobility; asking a patient with hemiparesis due to stroke or injury to take the paper in his or her hand and then to do two things with it, such as place it on the table and then on his or her lap because the patient obviously cannot fold it in half with one hand.

Reading. Have the patient look at a piece of paper on which you have printed in large, bold letters "CLOSE YOUR EYES" and ask them to do what it says. Score 1 point (total of 1 point) if the patient complies.

Writing. Provide the patient with a blank piece of paper (optional to have a line on the page) and ask him or her to write a sentence. To receive a point (score of 0 to 1), the sentence must have a subject and verb, and it must make sense. Correct grammar and punctuation are not needed. Skip this item for individuals who are unable to write because of motor or neurologic impairment (e.g., stroke, severe tremor, advanced Parkinson disease).

Construction. Provide the patient with a drawing of two intersecting pentagons, and ask him or her to copy it. To receive a point (possible score of 0 to 1), the copy must have all 10 angles in the pentagons, and the intersect must have four sides. Take into account the presence of tremor, abnormal motor movements, and hemiparesis. Skip this item for individuals who do not have the ability to draw because of motor impairment.

SCORING AND INTERPRETATION OF THE MINI-MENTAL STATE EXAMINATION

An individual's score should be reported as X out of 30, and it should include comment on which areas were missed. As was noted, some sensory and motor impairments allow a total possible score of between 25 and 27 only, in which case the dementia cutoff point can be adjusted down by the number of points skipped. In general, a score of 24 or below (out of 30) should raise questions about dementia, and it suggests the need for further testing. The author sometimes suspects cognitive impairment at scores of 25 or 26, depending on what was missed: someone who misses all three words on recall or who is not oriented at all to place may have underlying cognitive problems that warrant investigation.

 TIP

Remember, the MMSE is a screening test, not a gold standard, for determining dementia. You are not seeking to make a diagnosis with it but rather to identify someone with potential deficits in one or more key areas of cognition. Initially, think of the MMSE as a triage tool that helps you to plot a course for evaluation. After a diagnosis has been established, the MMSE can then serve to track the patient's course.

Normal scores for individuals with at least an eighth grade education range from 26 to 30. When the individual has less education, the normal scores may fall in a lower range (scores of 20 to 26), but more detailed neuropsychologic testing may then be warranted. Mild cognitive impairment is typically in the 20-point to 24-point range, moderate impairment is in the 10-point to 20-point range, and severe impairment generally falls below 10. In general, most individuals with AD lose anywhere from 2 to 4 points every year on the MMSE. Delirium and depression can drop a person's score dramatically, depending on how severely his or her degree of attention, concentration, and motivation is affected. Apathetic, uncooperative, and paranoid attitudes toward testing can also lower scores artificially. To gain a practical perspective on an individual's score, the clinician should not forget to look at his or her previous scores, clinical state, age, and education. When the clinician is not sure that he or she has scored one or more items correctly, he or she should be sure to document his or her questions or concerns along with the patient's score; he or she may consider adding a score range based on either including or excluding the items in question.

Clock Drawing Test

The CDT is a fascinating test in its simplicity, its ability to reveal deficits in a variety of domains, and the obviousness of its results. Looking at a misshapen clock, one intuitively knows whether someone's answer is wrong. The instructions for the CDT are simple: ask the patient to draw the face of a clock, place the numbers on it, and then draw in the hands to read 11:10 or alternatively 8:20. The logic behind why these two times are requested is that they force the patient to use both the left and right spatial fields and to maximize executive and frontal lobe function to assign 10 minutes to the number 2 (or 20 minutes to the number 4). The ability of an individual to complete this task correctly provides information on numerous domains of cognitive function, including memory, language comprehension, visuospatial and visuomotor skills, concentration, executive function, fine motor skills, mathematical ability, and visual fields. These skills rely on a variety of intact brain regions in both hemispheres, so injury to selective regions may well be reflected in the clock drawing.

Assessment of the clock drawing can be qualitative or quantitative, depending on the context in which it is being used. Many examiners simply present a copy of the drawing along with other clinical data and include commentary and interpretation of the results. Other examiners prefer to derive a numerical score for the drawing, so, over the years, researchers have developed a variety of methods to score and analyze the CDT. Perhaps the easiest method is found on the Mini-Cog—either the clock is correct in all its features (face, numbers, hands, and time) or it is incorrect, and the decision tree for likely dementia depends in part on this simple distinction. An equally simple but more quantitative scoring technique scores 1 point for the correct representation of the following four factors: (a) clock face drawn as circle, (b) numbers in correct positions, (c) all 12 positions included, and (d) hands in correct position. The 4-point scoring method and a more in-depth 10-point scoring technique are listed on Pocket Card A.4B in Appendix A.

Mini-Cog

The Mini-Cog is an extremely quick and simple screen that takes approximately 3 minutes to administer. It consists of a test for three-item recall and a clock drawing. Individuals are asked (a) to repeat three unrelated words (as in the MMSE), (b) to draw a clock (as in the CDT), and (c) to recall the three words. They are categorized as *probably demented* if they cannot recall any words and *probably not demented* if they recall all three. Individuals who recall only one or two words are categorized based on their CDT; they are considered *probably demented* if their clock is in any way abnormal and *probably not demented* if their clock is normally constructed. The method of categorization on the Mini-Cog is streamlined, and it eliminates the interpretation that inevitably follows the MMSE. Not only does the Mini-Cog serve as an excellent method of triage to identify individuals for more workup, but it also retains the CDT and the rich data that can be mined from its results.

Other screening tests

In addition to the MMSE, CDT, and Mini-Cog, several other screening tests for cognitive impairment warrant brief description. The *7-Minute Screen* consists of four parts: (a) a brief test of orientation, (b) a memory test using 16 picture cards, (c) a CDT, and (d) a test of verbal fluency that asks patients to name as many animals as they can in 60 seconds. The screening is supposed to take only 7 minutes, and it yields a composite score that indicates a high, low, or indeterminate probability of having AD. Although the test does a good job of identifying individuals with AD, it is not as effective with other forms of dementia. The *Cognitive Assessment Screening Test* (CAST) was designed for use in general physicians' offices. It consists of the following three parts: (a) screening questions and tasks that cover orientation, personal background, general knowledge, and visual construction skills; (b) mathematical and functional tests; and (c) 13 yes-or-no questions regarding the individual's history of cognitive problems. Although the CAST requires minimal examiner time and training, and, ostensibly, it can be filled out by patients sitting in a waiting room, it is limited to individuals with at least a high school education who have reasonably good skills to follow the directions to even complete the test. Having an examiner sit and lead the patient through the test probably takes 10 to 15 minutes.

The *Time and Change Test* is a relatively quick test that consists of two parts as follows: (a) the patient is asked to look at a clock set to 11:10 and tell the time and (b) the patient is asked to select one dollar in change from three quarters, seven dimes, and seven nickels. Failure to respond correctly to either task is a positive result for dementia. Although the Time and Change Test lacks extensive validation, it can be a useful bedside test in both outpatient and inpatient settings and it can easily be administered by most clinicians. It is limited only by an individual's knowledge of United States coinage. The *Blessed Information-Memory-Concentration Test* (BIMC) is another brief cognitive screening for dementia that predates the MMSE but that resembles it in form and content. The BIMC consists of 26 items that assess orientation, personal background, general knowledge, language, numerical sequencing, and memory. Two of the trickier items ask the patient to tell the dates of World Wars I and II, questions that become less familiar with successive generations. A shorter version of the BIMC, called the *Blessed Orientation-Memory-Concentration Test*, consists of six items from the BIMC. Finally, the *Short Test of Mental Status*, which is similar to the MMSE, assesses orientation, attention, recall, calculation, abstraction, visual construction, and knowledge and includes a clock drawing item. A guide to administering a cognitive screen can be found on Pocket Card A.4A (see also Table 5.5 for additional details).

Expanded Cognitive Screens

In some circumstances, a clinician may want to obtain a broader and more detailed cognitive screen without having to administer a full neuropsychologic test battery. An expanded cognitive screen could meet this goal, and it could also come in handy for individuals who, for one reason or another, will not likely return or cooperate with neuropsychologic testing (in other words, the clinician should use the opportunity he or she has to obtain as much information as possible). Several cognitive screening tests yield more information than the MMSE but take 20 to 45 minutes to administer. Each scale yields a composite score, as well as subscores for each domain or factor that is measured. These scales include the Mattis Dementia Rating Scale, the Neurobehavioral Cognitive Status Examination, the Neurobehavioral Rating Scale, and the Modified Mini-Mental State. The Alzheimer's Disease Assessment Scale, cognitive subscale, is a 1-hour test battery that is used to assess the efficacy of medications for AD. *References for several of the scales described in this chapter can be found in the suggested readings at the end of the book.*

5

The Dementia Workup III: Medical, Psychiatric, and Neuropsychologic Tests

> **Essential Concepts**
> • Laboratory testing and a brain scan are essential components of the dementia workup for identifying any treatable medical factors that are either causing or exacerbating cognitive impairment.
> • Neuropsychologic (NP) and functional testing build on the mental status examination and provide a clearer picture of the pattern, degree, and implications of cognitive impairment.

In addition to the medical and psychiatric history and examination, the three other basic components of the dementia workup are as follows: laboratory tests, a brain scan, and NP testing. Depending on the presentation, additional diagnostic procedures, such as a lumbar puncture and electroencephalography (EEG), may also be included in the workup. This chapter presents the rationale for each element.

LABORATORY TESTS

The essential laboratory tests in a standard dementia workup are listed in Table 5.1. These tests are especially important in the setting of acute changes in mental status or delirium because these states always have a medical cause (see Chapter 12 for more information on delirium and dementia). A complete blood count and urinalysis can help one rule out infection as an underlying factor in such cases. Other causes of both acute and more chronic cognitive impairment are abnormal electrolytes; alterations found on renal, thyroid, or liver function tests; and hypocalcemic and hypercalcemic states. Fasting glucose and hemoglobin A1c are used to identify and to track

TABLE 5.1. Standard Laboratory Tests in the Dementia Workup

Test	Potential cause of cognitive impairment
Complete blood count	Infection, anemia
Electrolytes	Hyponatremia, SIADH
Glucose	Diabetes mellitus, hypoglycemia
Renal function (BUN, creatinine)	Renal failure (uremia)
Calcium	Hypocalcemia or hypercalcemia, parathyroid disease
Thyroid function (TSH)	Hypothyroidism
Liver function	Hepatic encephalopathy
ESR	Vasculitis, unspecified inflammatory or malignant process
Vitamin B_{12}, folate	Vitamin B_{12} or folate deficiency
RPR/FTA/VDRL	Neurosyphilis
Urinalysis	Urinary tract infection, urosepsis, renal disease

Abbreviations: BUN, blood urea nitrogen; ESR, erythrocyte sedimentation rate; FTA, fluorescent treponemal antibody-absorption; RPR, rapid plasma reagent; SIADH, syndrome of inappropriate secretion of antidiuretic hormone; TSH, thyroid-stimulating hormone; VDRL, Venereal Disease Research Laboratory.

treatment of diabetes, a major cause of vascular dementia. Less common, but still important, causes of dementia that should be ruled out include deficiencies of vitamin B_{12} and folate.

Table 5.2 lists additional laboratory tests that might be ordered when the presentation of dementia has been precipitous, it occurs in a young and/or otherwise healthy individual, or it is associated with an unusual presentation. Many of these conditions are described in Chapter 11. For example, individuals who work in the mining or chemical industry may have been exposed to some heavy metals, and they can be tested accordingly. Suspicion of substance abuse always warrants conducting a urine drug screen. Individuals who have spent time hiking outdoors, especially in New England and the upper Midwest, should always be queried regarding tick bites and Lyme disease. Human immunodeficiency virus should always be included in the differential diagnosis because dementia can be an early symptom of this condition. A lumbar puncture is necessary for cerebrospinal fluid analysis when meningitis or encephalitis is suspected, and it is used to rule out neurosyphilis and multiple sclerosis as well.

TABLE 5.2. **Specialized Laboratory Tests**

Test	Potential cause of cognitive impairment
Drug screen	Substance abuse
Lyme titer	Lyme encephalopathy
Heavy metal screen	Mercury, lead, manganese, arsenic, cadmium, copper, and aluminum poisoning
HIV	HIV encephalopathy and/or AIDS dementia
Antinuclear antibody	Systemic lupus erythematosus
Cortisol	Adrenal disease (Addison or Cushing)
Ceruloplasmin	Wilson disease (abnormal copper metabolism)
Phosphorus	Parathyroid disease
Magnesium	Hypomagnesemia, alcohol dependence
Ammonia	Hepatic encephalopathy
Epstein–Barr virus	Viral encephalitis
Cytomegalovirus	Viral encephalitis
Long-chain fatty acids	Adrenoleukodystrophy
Arylsulfatase A	Metachromatic leukodystrophy
Porphobilinogen, ALA (24-h urine)	Acute intermittent porphyria
Cerebrospinal fluid	CNS infection, multiple sclerosis

Abbreviations: AIDS, acquired immunodeficiency syndrome; ALA, aminolevulinic acid; CNS, central nervous system; HIV, human immunodeficiency virus.

BRAIN SCANS

A brain scan is an essential feature of almost every dementia workup, and it serves to rule out the presence of structural lesions that may be causing cognitive impairment. Most clinicians opt to order a computed tomography (CT) scan of the brain because this is the quickest, easiest, and cheapest examination, and it is readily able to identify major strokes, bleeds, and masses. Conversely, magnetic resonance imaging (MRI) is superior to CT in identifying white matter lesions; smaller infarcts; subacute bleeding; and lesions in the brainstem, subcortical regions, and posterior fossa. Unlike CT, MRI can distinguish between white and gray matter, and no radiation exposure is involved. However, MRI is more expensive, less available, and more time-consuming, and it is not always well tolerated. With the use of MRI, the signal reception can be altered to produce T1-weighted images with startling tissue resolution or T2-weighted images with greater tissue contrast to identify some pathologic changes.

Regardless of the type of structural scan, some of the following anatomic changes in the brain are inevitably encountered with aging: generalized cerebral atrophy, increased ventricular size, and the presence of periventricular and subcortical calcifications and nonspecific "spots." These "spots" have been given many names in the literature (e.g., hyperintensities [as seen on MRI], unidentified bright objects, and leukoariosis), but all point to areas of likely neuronal injury due to one or more of the following factors: the effects of aging on the brain, chronic hypoperfusion, lacunar or atherosclerotic injury, gliosis, localized edema, and demyelination. The relevance of these spots to dementia is reviewed in Chapter 8 in the discussion of vascular dementia.

Of increasing importance to the dementia workup are functional brain scans, including positron emission tomography (PET) and single photon emission computed tomography (SPECT). Both PET and SPECT require the administration of radiolabeled isotopes to measure ongoing brain activity as a function of glucose metabolism or regional blood flow. Because of their complexity, however, the use of PET and SPECT scanning is, for the most part, limited to research institutions. Nevertheless, functional scanning will become more commonplace as technology advances and such scans prove more useful in the dementia workup.

ELECTROENCEPHALOGRAPHY

Although an EEG is not a routine part of the dementia workup, it can be useful if the following questions cannot be answered with the available history and the examination:

- Does the patient have an underlying seizure disorder?
- Is the condition dementia or delirium?
- Is the condition a true dementia or a pseudodementia (depression-associated dementia)?
- Does the individual have a sleep disorder?

In general, EEG activity in dementia is characterized by diffuse slowing of brain activity, with increased delta and theta frequency. EEG findings associated with aging, dementia, and related conditions are summarized in Table 5.3.

TABLE 5.3. Electroencephalography Findings in Dementia and Associated Conditions

Condition	EEG findings
Normal brain	Alpha activity during states of relaxation, beta activity during concentration and when anxious, and theta and delta activity during deep sleep
Normal aging	Minor decrease in mean frequency of alpha activity; increased theta activity, intermittent focal slowing
Seizure disorders	Paroxysmal bursts of spikes, slow waves, spike-and-wave complexes during seizures. Interictal EEG activity may appear normal, or it may show particular abnormal patterns
Focal lesions	EEG shows phase reversal, sharp waves or spikes over specific brain regions
Delirium	Loss of alpha activity; generalized theta and delta activity present. Triphasic waves seen in uremic and hepatic encephalopathy
Alzheimer disease	Background alpha activity slows and disorganizes as the disease progresses; increased presence of theta and delta activity
Vascular dementia	EEG changes resemble those in Alzheimer disease but appear unilateral or asymmetric, depending on the location of infarcts
Creutzfeldt–Jakob disease	Bursts of activity followed by minimal activity, called periodic complexes, associated with myoclonic jerks; bifrontal sharp waves or triphasic waves
Pseudodementia	EEG is normal, or it shows minimal slowing compared with EEG in Alzheimer disease

Abbreviation: EEG, electroencephalography.
From Kaufman DM. *Clinical neurology for psychiatrists.* Philadelphia: WB Saunders, 1995, with permission.

NEUROPSYCHOLOGIC TESTING

NP testing consists of the administration of a series of tests by a trained examiner to measure both the qualitative and quantitative aspects of a variety of cognitive skills. It builds on the mental status examination by providing greater detail across a broader range of cognitive domains. NP testing helps to characterize the patient's existing cognitive strengths and weaknesses, and it then correlates them with other aspects of brain structure and function. The resultant picture enables the clinician to construct the best possible diagnostic picture, and it provides a baseline against which the dementia can be tracked. The results also provide information on the individual's functional capacity so that an understanding of how his or her cognitive changes affect daily activities can be reached. This information can help the clinician sculpt the appropriate treatment interventions, including cognitive rehabilitation, counseling and psychotherapy, psychopharmacotherapy, and therapeutic activities. NP testing may also be part of a competency evaluation conducted to determine an individual's decision-making capacity.

Baseline NP testing should be ordered for most cases of early-stage and middle-stage dementia, as long as the patient can tolerate a 2-hour to 3-hour testing session. When the clinician is making a referral, he or she should always provide a summary of the dementia workup and should include diagnostic impressions and relevant questions to be answered by testing. For example, a clinician may want to rule out aphasia in a patient who has difficulty responding to questions, to evaluate for apathy versus depression, or to seek evidence of frontal lobe impairment. Guided by these diagnostic hypotheses and questions, the examiner can determine the most appropriate tests to administer. The examiner also adjusts the test battery to account for sensory, physical, cognitive, and behavioral limitations. For accurate testing, administering the test in the individual's most familiar language is best. Because testing often requires several hours, the examiner must also have a sense of what the patient can tolerate; he or she may then decide to break it up into several sessions. Subsequent interviews with family members, the analysis of test results, and the preparation of a report can take an additional several hours, thus underscoring how labor-intensive NP testing can be. The best examiners know how to put a patient at ease, to draw him or her out, and to provide support both during the testing and afterward when the results are reviewed. Over the course of the testing, examiners are sometimes the first clinicians to identify specific psychologic stresses and psychiatric disorders because they may spend more time with the patient than any other clinician does. Therefore, their reports should always be taken seriously, and their recommendations should be incorporated into the treatment plan.

 KEY POINT

Many clinicians postpone NP testing during the acute phase of a major depressive or psychotic episode. When the mood disorder or psychosis is more chronic, testing can actually serve a role in distinguishing impairment due to dementia from impairment secondary to the psychiatric condition.

CLINICAL VIGNETTE

Mr. Pardo, an 85-year-old Cuban immigrant fluent in Spanish and English, was hard of hearing, and he refused to wear a hearing aid. He was referred for NP testing to assess his memory impairment and irritable mood. Dr. Hernandez, the neuropsychologist, decided to administer the test battery in Spanish because Mr. Pardo's English was marginal, compared with his fluent Spanish. She also had him wear headphones connected to an amplifier to ensure that he heard all the questions. Because he presented in an irritable and impatient manner, she split the testing into three 1-hour sessions over the course of several weeks.

CLINICAL VIGNETTE

Mrs. Tetley, an 82-year-old woman with a long history of unspecified "mental problems," noncompliance with psychiatric care, and a recent onset of cognitive impairment, was referred for NP testing by her psychiatrist to determine whether dementia was present. Dr. Kinsey, the neuropsychologist, noted that Mrs. Tetley was quite talkative, sarcastic, and paranoid, with some obvious gaps in reasoning and judgment. Her memory was more or less intact. He spent most of the initial testing session listening to Mrs. Tetley's litany of complaints regarding her care at an assisted-living facility, and he offered to help her resolve a minor dispute with staff. At the second testing session, Dr. Kinsey administered several tests with a focus on frontal lobe function. He had Mrs. Tetley return for a third session, during which he administered the Rorschach Inkblot Test to assess her personality functioning. Overall, Mrs. Tetley's diagnostic picture leaned less toward a progressive dementia and more toward frontal lobe impairment in the setting of a personality disorder. Mrs. Tetley's psychiatrist was impressed by the results and decided to order a CT scan, which did demonstrate the presence of a frontal lobe meningioma.

Many neuropsychologists prefer to use a flexible approach to NP testing in which they select and modify tests from a variety of published batteries. Subsections of the Wechsler Adult Intelligence Scale–Revised and the Wechsler Memory Scales–Revised form the foundation of most NP testing because both contain subtests that are relevant to a variety of cognitive functions. All NP testing involves one of the brief cognitive screens cited in Chapter 4, of which the two most popular choices are the Mini-Mental State Examination (MMSE) and the Clock Drawing Test (CDT). More specific tests for evaluating frontal lobe impairment include the Wisconsin Card Sorting Test and the Trail-Making Test, Parts A and B. Some examiners administer a fixed battery of standardized tests, such as the Halstead–Reitan Neuropsychological Battery (HRNB) or the Luria–Nebraska Neuropsychological Battery. The Luria–Nebraska is less time-consuming than the HRNB, although, in their entireties, both test batteries may be too challenging for many older individuals with dementia. The examiner may instead decide to select subtests from each (the HRNB includes many classic NP subtests) or to use shorter versions. Personality assessment, including classic projective tests, such as the Rorschach Inkblot Test and the Thematic Apperception Test, is sometimes incorporated into NP testing. However, these tests require specialized training in administration, scoring, and interpretation, and they can be quite time-consuming.

FUNCTIONAL TESTING

NP assessment in dementia often includes functional testing, which attempts to identify how cognitive deficits translate into functional limitations that impact those skills often referred to as activities of daily living (ADLs) (e.g., dressing, grooming and hygiene, food preparation and feeding, operating appliances, driving, shopping, making change with money, writing checks). In addition to the neuropsychologist, a variety of clinicians may participate in making observations or conducting tests regarding daily function, including occupational and physical therapists, social workers, and recreational therapists. An important advantage to functional testing is that it helps to engage both the patient and caregivers in a discussion of both the patient's remaining strengths and weaknesses in the face of dementia.

CLINICAL VIGNETTE

Mr. Able was a 78-year-old farmer who lived in a rural part of the state that was 100 miles away from the Veterans Affairs hospital where he was sent for a dementia workup. He was found to have a moderate degree of cognitive impairment, likely due to Alzheimer disease. Still, he insisted on driving, arguing that he could easily navigate the country roads. NP testing indicated deficits in the cognitive ability to switch focus between completing sets of instructions on a single task, known as "set shifting." Translated into practical terms, this deficit indicated that, although Mr. Able may drive marginally well on a quiet country road during the middle of the day, he would be at much greater risk of having an accident or getting lost if he were driving on a busier road with competing stimuli, such as other cars, pedestrians, signal lights, and varying weather conditions. He was referred for a functional driving evaluation at the Veterans Affairs center, and he performed poorly on his reaction time, in line with other identified deficits.

Having to warn an individual of risky behaviors, especially driving, is never easy. Such information may pit family members or caregivers against the impaired individual or against each other—the last situation that any clinician wants to create. Functional testing can sometimes be key in clearly showing the family that the person's difficulty with particular tasks is not just *theoretical* but rather an *actuality*.

One of the most popular functional tests is the Instrumental Activities of Daily Living Scale (IADLS). The Instrumental

Activities of Daily Living Scale uses a caregiver interview to assess the following eight abilities that are often impaired early in the course of dementia: handling the telephone, finances, shopping, food preparation, housekeeping, laundry, transportation, and medication management. Other caregiver-rated functional tests include the Physical Self-Maintenance Scale, the Progressive Deterioration Scale, the Interview for Deterioration in Daily Living Activities in Dementia, and the Disability Assessment in Dementia Scale. (See "Suggested Readings" at the end of the text for specific citations.)

Because caregiver reports can sometimes be limited or biased, another approach to functional testing is to observe a model of ADL function. The Cognitive Performance Test asks an individual to perform six tasks in the clinic that mimic real-life situations and that can be observed and rated. Scoring is based on the Allen Cognitive Disability Theory that examines how functional performance is compromised by deficits in information processing and postulates six levels of functional disability ranging from profoundly disabled to normal. Narrative descriptions of each level provide a practical guide to what can be expected of an individual's performance both at home and in the community.

DEMENTIA STAGING

Both clinicians and researchers often use scales that rank an individual's dementia based on its stage of severity. Such a rating can serve several purposes as follows: (a) in research, it can be used to compare individuals and cohorts at a given time or over time; (b) in the clinic, it may help to predict current function, the relative need for social supports, and the disease course; and, (c) in long-term care, it can help the clinician anticipate the individual's psychosocial and nursing needs, including roommate and floor placement, activity selection, and the utility of particular rehabilitative therapies. The Global Deterioration Scale is a clinician-rated scale that provides seven stages of decline ranging from none to severe; these are listed in Table 5.4. The Brief Cognitive Rating Scale is rated by the clinician based on a structured interview with the patient and caregiver, and it assesses dementia on five axes, including orientation, concentration, memory (recent and past), and function. The Functional Assessment Staging is an extension of the function axis on the Brief Cognitive Rating Scale and provides a number of substages for individuals with more severe cogni-

TABLE 5.4. Global Deterioration Scale

Stage 1	Normal; no memory complaints and no evident cognitive impairment
Stage 2	Very mild; memory problem reported, but not evident in clinical interview
Stage 3	Mild impairment in memory, concentration, and occupational performance
Stage 4	Moderate impairment in memory, knowledge retrieval, and complex tasks
Stage 5	Moderate to severe impairment in both recent and remote memory, frequent disorientation to time and place, and impairment in activities of daily living that indicates need for caregiver assistance
Stage 6	Severe cognitive impairment with inability to tend to activities of daily living without assistance
Stage 7	Very severe impairment in cognition, language, and motor skills, progressing to a less functional, vegetative state

Modified from Reisberg B, Ferris SH, de Leon MJ, et al. The Global Deterioration Scale for assessment of primary degenerative dementia. *Am J Psychiatry* 1982;139: 1136–1139, with permission.

tive decline. Two other scales are the Functional Activities Questionnaire, a clinician-based instrument that assigns a stage from 1 (*normal*) to 7 (*severely incapacitated* in terms of ADL function), and the Clinical Dementia Rating Scale, a structured interview with both the patient and caregiver that rates individuals from 0 (*healthy*) to 4 (*profound*) and 5 (*terminal*) based on six cognitive and functional domains.

 TIP

The bedside NP examination is a condensed form of the dementia workup; it consists of a brief mental status examination followed by a cognitive screen, preferably the MMSE and the CDT (Table 5.5). It is useful for rapid cognitive assessment with medically compromised individuals and in busy clinics. Although the MMSE and CDT provide most of the data, additional information on specific cognitive skills, such as frontal lobe function, can be quickly obtained from the Trail-Making Test, the complex picture test, or other tests that a neuropsychologist can suggest.

TABLE 5.5. Bedside Neuropsychologic Examination

Memory	Immediate: repetition of three objects (MMSE)
	Recent: recall of three objects (MMSE)
	Remote: recall of past events
Aphasia	Comprehension: ability to follow simple commands (MMSE and CDT)
	Expressive: repetition of "no ifs, ands, or buts" (MMSE)
	Listen for missed or mispronounced words, nonsensical words
	Naming (anomia): ask patient to identify common objects (MMSE)
Apraxia	Constructional: ability to copy pentagons on MMSE, clock face on CDT, or simple objects (outline of a cross or a key)
	Ideomotor: ability to demonstrate how to comb hair, brush teeth, or hammer nail
Agnosia	Prosopagnosia: impaired recognition of familiar faces (e.g., family)
	Astereognosis: impaired recognition of familiar objects via tactile exploration
	Finger agnosia: ask patient to identify finger by touch
Executive function	Ability to plan and sequence steps of making clock (CDT)
	Ability to reproduce rhythm with finger tapped out by examiner
	Ability to mimic sequence using same hand: (a) slap fist on table, (b) open fist and slap side of hand on table, (c) slap palm on table
Function	Four IADL score: ask caregiver whether patient needs assistance in these areas: (a) money management, (b) medication management, (c) telephone use, and (d) traveling. Suspect dementia with increased need for assistance

Abbreviations: CDT, Clock Drawing Test; IADL, Instrumental Activities of Daily Living Scale; MMSE, Mini-Mental State Examination.

PRESENTING THE OVERALL FINDINGS

After the dementia workup is complete, the clinician must propose a diagnosis and a treatment plan. Presenting the results as clearly and consistently as possible and avoiding vague or conflicting diagnoses is important for both the patient and family. The last few paragraphs of the NP report usually suggest diagnoses that may or may not be in agreement with the clinician's thinking. If a discrepancy is present (i.e., the neuropsychologist suggests a diagnosis of Alzheimer disease but the clinician is convinced it is dementia with Lewy bodies), a discussion with the examiner is warranted. NP test reports can sometimes be confusing; after all, without understanding the details of each test, including the normative scores, and the correlations between test results, brain function, and performance in the real world, incorporating the results into diagnostic impressions and recommendations can be difficult. Therefore, clinicians must have a rudimentary understanding of the purpose and nature of the tests, and they should communicate in person with the examiner to gain further insight into the selection of tests and the overall meaning of the results.

The clinician should take time to educate both the patient and family about the diagnosis and its expected course, and he or she should emphasize both the strengths and weaknesses of the patient's current state. Excessively technical or quantitative descriptions should be avoided, but the data should be used to support the diagnosis and they should be translated into practical implications for daily function. Functional test results help in that regard. The clinician may recommend additional medical or psychiatric workups for residual questions if he or she suspects a reversible cause or he or she may continue with treatment recommendations, including preventive measures against further cognitive decline, attention to safety issues, treatment for a behavioral problem or psychiatric condition, assistance with ADLs, increased therapeutic activities and social stimulation, better monitoring at home, or placement in a more structured setting. When these recommendations have been formulated, documented, and communicated to the patient, family, and caregivers, the dementia workup is complete. The next step is the implementation of the recommendations, a topic that is covered throughout the remainder of the book.

DEMENTIA SUBTYPES

Alzheimer Disease:
Definition and Diagnosis

> **Essential Concepts**
> - Alzheimer disease (AD) is the most common form of dementia, representing approximately 70% of all cases and afflicting four to five million Americans.
> - Current research points to the following two factors as potential causes of AD: extraneuronal deposition of β-amyloid and intraneuronal destabilization of tau protein.
> - Most cases of AD begin after 65 years of age, and they are not associated with known genetic causes. Risk factors include advancing age, menopause, brain injury, lower education, and the presence of the apolipoprotein E4 (APOE4) genetic allele.
> - The diagnosis of AD relies on patient history and neuropsychologic testing. Biomarkers and genetic testing may only marginally increase diagnostic certainty.

Although medical knowledge of dementia has existed for centuries, the modern-day knowledge of the most common form of dementia began slightly more than 100 years ago. In late 1901, a 51-year-old woman in Germany was brought to a psychiatric hospital after a several-month history of progressive memory impairment and behavioral disturbances, including angry outbursts and paranoid ideation. For the next 4 years, she was followed by a psychiatrist who charted her downward course of increasing cognitive impairment; psychiatric disturbances; and, ultimately, a vegetative state before death. After her death, her stalwart psychiatrist, who had been unable to determine an exact diagnosis throughout her long course, was finally able to view the actual brain tissue. The results were startling—the brain cells were crowded and blotted out by brown-stained clumps of material, and the cells themselves were overrun by tangles of dark fibrils that appeared to have destroyed other cellular components. This dedicated and relentless physician, Dr. Alois Alzheimer, was looking at what clinicians now know as plaques and tangles, the pathologic hallmarks of the disease that he first wrote about and that today bears his name.

At this time, AD is recognized as the most common form of dementia, and it accounts for, either alone or in part, as many as 70% of all cases. It afflicts an estimated 4 to 5 million persons in the United States. After the age of 65, the prevalence rate doubles every 5 years such that, although fewer than 5% of individuals who are 65 years of age have AD, nearly 50% of individuals who are 85 years and older are affected. Because this most vulnerable age group is also one of the fastest growing segments of the population, AD will afflict at least 10 million persons in the United States by the year 2030, barring any major advances in the prevention of the disease. The realization that AD is the fourth leading cause of death in the United States is sobering. Not surprisingly, the social and economic burdens are staggering; the annual costs of AD to the United States economy are estimated to be as high as $100 billion, making it the third most expensive disease after cancer and heart disease. The annual caregiving costs per patient for mild AD average roughly $18,000, a figure that doubles in the severe stages of the disease. The total expenditures for an individual over the typical 8-year to 10-year course of the disease may be as high as $200,000.

Aside from these numbers, the most daunting aspect of AD lies in its very nature as a progressive and incurable disorder. Until approximately 10 years ago, AD was also relatively untreatable, which may account for the reactions that many individuals and their families demonstrate in its early stages: the denial of illness, covering up the individual's deficits, or fatalism over its course. Perhaps these reactions also account for the fact that fewer than half of those individuals in the United States who have AD actually have been clinically diagnosed with the condition and that fewer than one-fourth of the total receive specific treatment. This is true despite the fact that many obvious benefits to early diagnosis exist (see Chapter 1) and even though effective pharmacologic treatments for the symptoms of AD have been on the market for more than 10 years (see Chapter 7).

WHAT IS ALZHEIMER DISEASE?

AD is a cortical dementia characterized by a slow, progressive loss of cognitive function that typically lasts for 8 to 12 years (range of 5 to 20 years) and culminates in a vegetative state and then death. The clinical signs of AD typically manifest in later life, although the pathologic features may begin much earlier. AD has been classified by age of onset (early or late) and by the presence or absence of an inheritance pattern (familial versus sporadic). Early-onset AD, which accounts for only 5% to 10% of all cases of AD, presents before the age of 65 years and typically has a relatively rapid course. Late-onset AD, conversely, accounts for the other 90% to 95% of cases and has an onset after the age of 65. All of the known cases of familial AD have had an early onset, and they have been traced to specific chromosomal mutations. Sporadic AD tends to have a later age at onset, and it is associated with some degree of genetic susceptibility. Further research may eventually identify patterns of inheritance in sporadic AD, but these will be more difficult to recognize and they will certainly entail an interaction between genetic and environmental factors. Genetic factors are reviewed in more detail in the section on AD risk factors.

DIAGNOSTIC CRITERIA

Currently, the following two sets of diagnostic criteria are most commonly used for AD: the *Diagnostic and Statistical*

TABLE 6.1. *Diagnostic and Statistical Manual of Mental Disorders, Fourth Edition, Text Revision,* **Criteria for Dementia of the Alzheimer Type**

A. The development of multiple cognitive deficits manifested by both memory impairment and one or more of the following: aphasia, apraxia, agnosia, and disturbances in executive functioning

B. The cognitive deficits represent a decline from previous functioning and cause significant impairment in social or occupational functioning

C. The course is characterized by gradual onset and continuing cognitive decline

D. The cognitive deficits are not due to other central nervous system, systemic, or substance-induced conditions that cause progressive deficits in memory and cognition

E. The disturbance is not better accounted for by another psychiatric disorder

From American Psychiatric Association *Diagnostic and statistical manual of mental disorders,* fourth edition, text revision. Washington, D.C.: American Psychiatric Association, 2000, with permission.

Manual of Mental Disorders, Fourth Edition, Text Revision (DSM-IV-TR) criteria and the National Institute of Neurological and Communicative Disorders and Stroke–Alzheimer's Disease and Related Disorders Association (NINDS-ADRDA) criteria. These are listed in Tables 6.1 and 6.2, respectively. The critical aspect of AD present in both sets of criteria is the progressive and global nature of cognitive impairment. As this book outlines throughout, the other major forms of dementia tend to involve more specific areas of impairment, and they generally have a more rapid or a less predictable course. NINDS-ADRDA criteria are unique in accounting for the probability of the diagnosis.

TABLE 6.2. National Institute of Neurological and Communicative Disorders and Stroke–Alzheimer's Disease and Related Disorders Association Criteria for Definite, Probable, and Possible Alzheimer Disease

Definite AD	Meets criteria for probable AD and has histopathologic evidence of AD via autopsy or biopsy
Probable AD	Dementia established by clinical and neuropsychologic examination and involves (a) progressive deficits in two or more areas of cognition, including memory, (b) onset between the ages of 40 and 90 years, and (c) absence of systemic or other brain diseases capable of producing a dementia syndrome, including delirium
Possible AD	A dementia syndrome with an atypical onset, presentation, or progression and without a known etiology
	Any comorbid diseases capable of producing dementia are not believed to be the cause
Unlikely AD	A dementia syndrome with any of the following: sudden onset, focal neurologic signs, or seizures or gait disturbance early in the course of the illness

Abbreviation: AD, Alzheimer disease.

From McKhann G, Drachman D, Folstein M, et al. Clinical diagnosis of Alzheimer's disease: report of the NINCDS–ADRDA work group under the auspices of Department of Health and Human Services Task Force on Alzheimer's Disease. *Neurology* 1984;34:939–944, with permission.

THE COURSE OF ALZHEIMER DISEASE

AD typically begins with subtle changes in memory and orientation, including frequent forgetfulness, difficulty with complex daily tasks (e.g., balancing a checkbook, planning events or projects), word-finding difficulty, and lapses in the recognition of persons or places. This early stage may last several years, and it can be indistinguishable at times from the more mild states of cognitive impairment due to medication side effects; medical or psychiatric illness; or syndromes, such as age-associated memory impairment or mild cognitive impairment (see Chapter 1).

As AD progresses, the cognitive deficits worsen, becoming more global, and the incidence of comorbid psychiatric disturbances, such as anxiety, depression, apathy, agitation, and psychosis, is increased. Individual function declines to the point that independent living becomes too hazardous, and individuals must rely on caregivers and structured living arrangements. By 8 to 10 years into the illness, the early disturbances in memory, language (aphasia), motor abilities (apraxia), and recognition (agnosia) progress to severe states, rendering an individual totally dependent on caregivers. In the terminal phase of AD, the afflicted individuals are usually incoherent or completely mute; they are unable to recognize their surroundings and close family members; and, ultimately, they are incapable of walking, feeding themselves, or even participating in simple activities. The behavioral problems may begin to taper off, but they are overridden by a collapse of function and an increasing incidence of poor feeding, malnutrition, injuries from falls and unsafe behaviors, and pressure sores caused by inactivity. Death does not result from the pathologic effects of AD itself but rather from associated infection, dehydration, injury, or other medical illnesses.

CLINICAL VIGNETTE

Mrs. Soble was a 75-year-old retired real estate broker with a history of mild depression and migraine headaches. Her daughter began to notice some mild forgetfulness in her mother, such as not remembering the content of recent phone conversations. She also noticed that her mother was more irritable at times and that she was less sociable with her friends. She attributed this to increased depression and urged

her mother to see her psychiatrist. Dr. Bergan agreec
Mrs. Soble seemed depressed, and she restarted her c
selective serotonin reuptake inhibitor antidepressant that r
previously helped. Despite some improvement in her moo
Mrs. Soble continued to demonstrate forgetfulness with fre
quent bouts of disorientation when driving. She had to call
her daughter on several occasions to get assistance in returning home. Twelve months after first noticing these changes,
Mrs. Soble's daughter took her to her physician for a full medical workup, which was unrevealing. Mrs. Soble was referred
to a dementia clinic, where the evaluation suggested a diagnosis of probable AD.

Over the course of the next year, the symptoms progressed
to the point that Mrs. Soble could no longer safely drive, and
she was increasingly unable to balance her checkbook or to
manage her small house. In the third year of illness, Mrs.
Soble moved into an independent living facility, but, within 3
months, she was asked to leave because of her inability to
manage her medications safely and to maintain her apartment. Her daughter moved her into an assisted-living facility
where the additional structure and an aide for 5 hours every
day allowed her to maintain some degree of independence.
Over the next 2 years, however, Mrs. Soble's memory continued to decline, as did her ability to orient herself in the building and to recognize staff members. She became dependent
on her daughter to manage all her affairs. She also demonstrated paranoid concerns that her aides were trying to steal
from her, and, on two occasions, she barricaded herself in her
apartment. Her psychiatrist increased her antidepressant and
added an antipsychotic medication to calm her and to treat
her paranoid delusions.

In the sixth year of her illness, Mrs. Soble fell in her apartment and broke her hip. She became delirious after the hip
replacement, and, after some improvement in her mental status, she was admitted to a skilled nursing facility for rehabilitation. Because of her pronounced cognitive impairment and
periods of combativeness with staff, Mrs. Soble was trans-
ferred to a dementia unit at a long-term care facility instead of
returning to the assisted-living facility. By the seventh year of
her illness, Mrs. Soble was able to recognize only her daughter; she was unable to communicate well because of word-
finding difficulty. By the eighth year, she was completely
dependent on the staff for hygiene and dressing, although,
with prompting, she could still feed herself. Over the course
of the year, she fell several times, becoming wheelchair bound.

..ghout the ninth year, Mrs. Soble spent most of her day
..g in her wheelchair or lying in bed, with minimal verbal
..munication. She no longer recognized her daughter. She
..gan losing weight, and she became malnourished due to a
..oor appetite and mild dysphagia. In the tenth year, Mrs.
Soble developed an aspiration pneumonia and stopped eating.
After 2 weeks in a vegetative state, she died.

The course of Mrs. Soble's illness illustrates the slow and
progressive course of AD, which begins with memory dysfunction and evolves over time to involve the loss of multiple cognitive skills; changes in behavior and personality; and the loss
of basic bodily functions, ultimately culminating in death.

THE STORY OF ALZHEIMER DISEASE

Overview

With aging, every brain shows the same pathologic changes
as those that cripple the brains of individuals with AD—the
loss of neurons with subsequent shrinking or atrophy of
brain tissue, widened ventricles, and pathologic collections of
cellular debris known as neuritic plaques and neurofibrillary
tangles. One age-related cause for this neuronal damage in
both normal and AD brains may be oxidative stress, in which
the accumulation of reactive oxygen species called free radicals damage the DNA and other cellular components. In AD,
however, a dramatic acceleration and augmentation of this
process occurs, such that brain structure and function slowly
and steadily erode, producing the clinical symptoms that
have been described. A schematic of the entire pathologic
process of AD as it is currently understood is illustrated in
Figure 6.1.

Amyloid and Tau

Most scientists now believe that the story of AD begins with
the abnormal buildup of *β-amyloid protein* in the brain. Amyloid originates from part of a larger protein called the amyloid
precursor protein (APP), which is normally found in the cell
membranes of neurons throughout the brain. The exact role of
APP has not yet been determined, but the belief is that a pro-
tease enzyme called α-secretase normally metabolizes it. In
AD, however, the metabolism of APP is altered by two other

```
┌─────────────────────────────────────────────────┐
│                 DISEASE TRIGGERS                │
│          Genetic mutations or risk factors      │
│          Other risk factors, unknown factors    │
└─────────────────────────────────────────────────┘
```

↓

```
┌─────────────────────────────────────────────────┐
│            NEURITIC PLAQUE FORMATION            │
│          Extracellular Beta-Amyloid Deposition  │
│       APP –( beta / gamma secretase)→ Beta-Amyloid │
│                                                 │
│          NEUROFIBRILLARY TANGLE FORMATION       │
│        Intracellular Cytoskeleton Destabilization │
│   Tau protein hyperphosphorylation → Paired Helical Filaments │
└─────────────────────────────────────────────────┘
```

↓

```
┌─────────────────────────────────────────────────┐
│                  NEUROTOXICITY                  │
│   Entorhinal cortex, hippocampus, basal forebrain first │
│          Then other regions of cerebral cortex  │
└─────────────────────────────────────────────────┘
```

↓

```
┌─────────────────────────────────────────────────┐
│                  INFLAMMATION                   │
│          Response to beta-amyloid deposition    │
│             Accelerated cerebral atrophy        │
└─────────────────────────────────────────────────┘
```

↓

```
┌─────────────────────────────────────────────────┐
│              CHOLINERGIC DEFICITS               │
└─────────────────────────────────────────────────┘
```

↓

```
┌─────────────────────────────────────────────────┐
│            CLINICAL SYMPTOMS OF AD              │
└─────────────────────────────────────────────────┘
```

FIG. 6.1. The development of Alzheimer disease (AD).
Abbreviation: APP, amyloid precursor protein.

enzymes, β-secretase and γ-secretase (also referred to as β-site or γ-site APP cleaving enzyme [BACE and GACE]), which cleave APP, producing a protein fragment of 42 amino acids. This abnormal form of amyloid is referred to as β-amyloid. Whether one or both secretase enzymes are required to form the β-amyloid fragment is unclear. Once β-amyloid is formed, however, it has a tendency to accumulate into insoluble sheets (called β-pleated sheets) that build up in the brain in the spaces between neurons and in small blood vessels.

Insoluble β-amyloid deposits are problematic in two ways. First, they are neurotoxic, leading to the death of surrounding neurons. Second, the β-amyloid deposits act as foreign bodies in the brain, inducing an inflammatory response that causes further neuronal damage and death. Activated leukocytes and microglial cells begin to release the chemical mediators of inflammation, in turn activating the surrounding astrocyte cells. The pathologic result is a lesion or plaque—the infamous senile or neuritic plaque—consisting of a dense core of amyloid protein sheets surrounded by damaged and dead axons, dendrites, and glial cells (microglia and astrocytes). The belief that this entire process causes AD is referred to as the *amyloid cascade hypothesis*. Although an incredible amount of research has implicated this process, whether amyloid is the cause of AD or a byproduct of some other undiscovered cause is not clear.

At the same time that plaques are forming, a parallel process inside the neuronal cell bodies is wreaking havoc by destroying the cell's main support structure (or cytoskeleton) and the transport system composed of microtubules. A protein called *tau* that stabilizes the microtubule architecture becomes hyperphosphorylated, causing strands of it to wind around each other in what are called *paired helical filaments*. These filaments are unable to stabilize the microtubule system; instead, they begin to aggregate into the clumps referred to as *neurofibrillary tangles*. Deprived of its inner structural support and system of intracellular communication, the cell body is no longer able to function normally.

As the plaques and tangles proliferate, a progressive loss of neurons and their supporting glial cells occurs, such that a gross examination of the AD brain reveals marked cortical atrophy with widened sulci and ventricles. A closer inspection of the brain tissue indicates that the following key brain regions are affected successively during the course of AD: the entorhinal cortex; the hippocampus; the basal forebrain; and, eventually, general cortical regions. Both the entorhinal cortex and the hippocampus, which are located adjacent to one another in the temporal lobes, are critical to memory formation. Functional scanning has found that deterioration in these structures is an early indicator of AD. The loss of neurons in these structures probably accounts for the early symptoms of short-term memory impairment in AD. The basal forebrain, particularly the nucleus basalis of Meynert, contains numerous cell bodies that produce and transmit messages throughout the brain via the neurotransmitter *acetylcholine*.

The *cholinergic hypothesis* suggests that the resultant deficiency in acetylcholine, and hence in cholinergic function, is responsible for the clinical symptoms of AD. One experimental model supporting this hypothesis has demonstrated that the intravenous administration of anticholinergic drugs (e.g., scopolamine) can induce impairments in memory and cognitive function that are similar to the symptoms of AD. Other research has linked anticholinergic load in the body with an increased risk of delirium.

As the disease progresses, the neuronal loss becomes more pronounced in the temporal, parietal, occipital, and frontal cortices. These changes account for the cardinal features of the disease—aphasia, apraxia, agnosia, and executive dysfunction. In addition, damage to the brain regions that regulate behavior, emotional expression, and neurovegetative function (e.g., sleeping, eating, motivation), including the amygdala, locus ceruleus, and raphe nucleus, occurs. The latter two nuclei regulate the synthesis and the release of the neurotransmitters norepinephrine and serotonin, respectively. Abnormal alterations in one or both chemicals in the brain may account for the high prevalence of depression and behavioral problems in AD.

WHO IS AT RISK OF DEVELOPING ALZHEIMER DISEASE?

Numerous risk factors for AD exist, many of which can be tied into the pathologic scheme just described. Risk factors are summarized in Tables 6.3 and 6.4.

Age

Given that prevalence rates double every 5 years after age 65 so that 40% to 50% of the community older than 85 years is afflicted with AD, advanced age is the most dramatic risk factor for AD. As was noted, the oxidative stress caused by free radicals may be one age-related element, although this certainly is not the only, nor the most influential, one.

Genes

Genetic risk factors constitute some of the most widely studied aspects of AD, and these have proven to be the most informative in the search for a cause. Having a first-degree

TABLE 6.3. Risk Factors for Alzheimer Disease

Increased age	
Female gender	
Postmenopausal state (loss of estrogen)	
Genetic factors:	Family history in first-degree relative; Mutations on chromosomes 1, 14, 21; possibly on 10, 12, as well; APOE4 allele (chromosome 19); Trisomy 21 (Down syndrome)
Brain injury:	Head trauma with loss of consciousness, Vascular damage due to disease
Disease:	Hypertension, hypercholesterolemia, diabetes mellitus, atherosclerotic disease
Major depressive disorder	
Mild cognitive impairment	
Lower intelligence	
Less education	
Lifestyle:	Less physical, social, and intellectual activity
Smaller head and brain size	

relative with AD, such as a parent or a sibling, increases the risk of getting AD by approximately three and a half times. The risk is greatest if a sibling is affected, and it increases with the number of affected relatives. Identical (or monozygotic) twins have a 50% concordance rate for AD.

Early-onset AD, which includes all familial subtypes, has been traced to genetic mutations on chromosomes 1, 14, and 21, all of which are associated with the increased production of β-amyloid. The mode of inheritance in all three cases is autosomal dominant, meaning that a person needs only one copy of the gene from a parent to be affected. Scientists have proposed that the presenilin 1 gene on chromosome 14 and the presenilin 2 gene on chromosome 1 may actually be equivalent to β-secretase and γ-secretase, the enzymes responsible for creating β-amyloid in the first place. Approximately 40% of early-onset cases are linked to chromosome 14, whereas those cases linked to chromosome 1 are encountered in a small group of families who are the descendants of

TABLE 6.4. Genetic Risk Factors for Alzheimer Disease

Type of AD	Chromosome	Gene	Effects
Early onset (5%–10%)	1	PS2	Increases β-amyloid; PS2 may be a secretase enzyme
	14	PS1	Increases β-amyloid; PS1 may be a secretase enzyme
	21	APP	Increases APP and β-amyloid
Late onset (90%–95%)	19	πAPOE	Presence of E4 allele increases susceptibility to AD, homozygotes >> heterozygotes
	10	LOAD	Late-onset AD gene, may impair β-amyloid clearance
	12	A2M	Uncertain
Family history	?	?	Risk 3.5 times greater if first-degree relative affected

Abbreviations: AD, Alzheimer disease; A2M, $α_2$ macroglobulin; APOE, apolipoprotein E; APP, amyloid precursor protein; LOAD, late-onset Alzheimer disease; PS1, presenilin 1; PS2, presenilin 2.

From Tanzi RE. A genetic dichotomy model for the inheritance of Alzheimer's disease and common age-related disorders. *J Clin Invest* 1999;104:1175–1179; and Tanzi RE, Blacker D. Genetic screening in Alzheimer's disease. *Generations* 2000;24:58–63.

German immigrants to the United States from the Volga River Valley. The other early-onset genetic mutation has been traced to a gene on chromosome 21 that may code for APP. This may well explain why individuals with Down syndrome who have three copies of chromosome 21 (trisomy 21) face the inevitable development of AD pathology (although not necessarily its clinical symptoms) by their 40s.

Late-onset AD, which encompasses the sporadic forms of the disease, has a more complex genetic picture than does early-onset AD. Instead of being associated with specific genetic mutations that may cause the disease, late-onset AD is associated with the APOE gene variants on chromosome 19 that, in part, determine the susceptibility for developing the disease. APOE is involved in the lipid metabolism that assists in myelination and neuronal membrane repair. It is found in both neurons and glial cells and in increased amounts in neuritic plaques. The isoforms of APOE are encoded by three alleles labeled E2, E3, and E4, of which E3 is the most common. Everyone inherits one allele from each parent, producing the following six possible genotypes: E2/E2, E2/E3, E2/E4, E3/E3, E3/E4, and E4/E4. E3/E3 is the most common genotype; it is seen in 60% of the population. The APOE2 and APOE3 alleles may actually be protective against AD, whereas the APOE4 allele confers a much higher risk of the disease, with a younger age at onset and a worse course.

Overall, 50% of late-onset cases of AD have the E4 allele; having one copy (heterozygote) increases the risk of developing AD by three times, whereas having two copies (homozygote) increases risk by five to 15 times, depending on age. By the age of 80, 90% of APOE4 homozygotes will have developed AD, compared with nearly 50% of APOE4 heterozygotes and 20% of individuals without an APOE4 allele. Women with the E4 allele have a much higher risk of contracting AD. However, even having both APOE4 alleles does not guarantee that the individual will develop AD, a clear indication that other factors are involved.

Recently, several research groups found a possible site on chromosome 10 that may work by elevating the levels of β-amyloid in the brain. This gene is independent of the APOE gene, and it may account for many of the individuals with AD who lack the APOE4 mutation. Scientists initially labeled the gene *LOAD* for *late-onset AD*. Finally, the gene for α_2-macroglobulin found on chromosome 12 may also be involved in increasing an individual's susceptibility to AD. All of the genetic risk factors for AD are summarized in Table 6.4.

Estrogen

Women have a greater risk of developing AD, even after taking into account the fact that they live longer than men. This difference may be due to the loss of estrogen after menopause and of its proposed benefits on cerebral function, including promotion of neural growth and development, reduction of plasma levels of APOE, antiinflammatory and antioxidant effects, increase of cerebral blood flow, and memory enhancement due to improved central cholinergic function.

Cognitive Reserve

The amount of brain and the number of synaptic connections may also influence AD risk because individuals with a smaller head and brain size, less intelligence, and less formal education earlier in life are at increased risk for the development of AD. Some researchers have suggested that all of these factors contribute to the development of a cognitive reserve in the brain that serves to reduce the risk and/or blunt the symptoms of AD. Some evidence of these risk factors has been found in the now famous Nun Study, an ongoing longitudinal study of AD in which an order of nuns have agreed to be studied as they age and then to donate their brains after death. By reviewing the essays written by the nuns in early adulthood when they applied to the order, the researchers found that lower linguistic ability (as measured by the degree of grammatical complexity and the idea density in sentences) was associated with higher rates of AD. The study raises the question of whether early preclinical pathologic changes in the brains of those who later developed AD subtly limited their intelligence and academic attainment or whether individuals with lower intelligence or less education had lifestyles that increased the risk of AD. Perhaps both factors interact in some as yet undetermined manner.

Brain Damage

Any process that causes significant brain damage, even earlier in life, can increase the risk of AD. This includes head trauma with loss of consciousness and vascular damage from a variety of interrelated causes, such as stroke, atherosclerotic disease, hypertension, hypercholesterolemia, and diabetes mellitus. In general, head injury may increase the risk of AD by two to four times, depending on the severity of the injury. The belief is that brain injury may trigger the production of β-amyloid; in fact, several studies have found increased β-amyloid in the areas of previous trauma. Other disease states associated with brain damage and an increased risk of AD include major depression (especially when it is associated with transient cognitive impairment or pseudodementia) and mild cognitive impairment. One possible explanation is that the elevated levels of cortisol associated with depression may be toxic to neurons in the hippocampus. The damage associated with mild cognitive impairment is not clear, but, per year, 15% of the affected individuals progress to AD.

Lifestyle

Interestingly enough, research has found that individuals with less physical, social, and mental activity have higher rates of AD. Conceivably, less physical activity may be associated with an increased prevalence of vascular risk factors that serve to increase the risk of AD. Similarly, less social and intellectual activity may be associated with a smaller cognitive reserve and thus less protection against AD pathology. Increased social isolation has also been associated with increased dementia. One study in Sweden interviewed 1,200 people 75 years of age and older, with follow-up 3 years later. Results showed that those who lived alone, had no friends, or had a poor relationship with their children were 60% more likely to develop dementia.

DIAGNOSIS

Even without knowing anything about a given patient with dementia, clinicians do know through epidemiologic studies that 70% of all cases involve AD. In other words, even if one guesses at a diagnosis of AD, he or she is apt to be correct. At present, however, the only way to make a diagnosis of AD with 100% certainty is to examine brain tissue for the presence of plaques and tangles. Obviously, this is not a realistic approach in the majority of patients. The diagnosis of AD, however, is by no means guesswork, and making a solid diagnosis with 90% to 95% accuracy is possible. Research is on the verge of breakthroughs that will increase this certainty even more. The diagnostic workup for AD involves all the components outlined in Chapters 1 through 5; in this chapter, the focus is on several specific findings that point more to AD than to another type of dementia.

TIP

Patients and caregivers often, and not surprisingly, want as much diagnostic certainty as possible. You will be asked frequently "Does he or she have Alzheimer disease?" Although providing a clear answer to a family's question is important, do not rush to judgment. Many individuals may appear to have AD, but observation over time does not support the diagnosis. You do not want to provide a diagnosis with such a bleak course without having all of the available information. Conversely, do not cover up the possibility of AD, and give false hope to patients and families. However, until a diagnosis for AD can be made with 100% certainty, you will always be in the position of having to make an educated guess.

History and Examination

The history of the dementia is the first diagnostic clue; a slowly progressive decline in cognitive function, starting with memory impairment and increasingly involving aphasia, apraxia, agnosia, and executive dysfunction, almost always points to AD. If persistent focal impairment or noticeable improvement is observed, then the case is almost certainly not AD. The diagnosis can be more difficult when symptoms consistent with AD overlap with vascular risk factors; a history of stroke; or other diseases known to cause cognitive impairment, such as Parkinson disease. Sometimes, early AD is associated with pronounced personality change, behavioral disturbances, depression, or psychosis (see Chapters 12 through 14 for more information). The neurologic examination is often unrevealing, and it cannot confirm the diagnosis. In the early and middle stages of AD, no characteristic findings are present, whereas the later stages of AD may involve increased motor dysfunction with unsteady gait, dysarthria and dysphagia, and myoclonus.

Neuroimaging

AD has been associated with a number of neuroradiographic findings. Structural computed tomography and magnetic resonance imaging (MRI) typically reveal progressive cerebral atrophy that is especially prominent in the hippocampus. If possible, the diagnostic scan should try to highlight and enlarge the hippocampus to determine the degree of atrophy. In AD, evidence of vascular damage in the brain caused by strokes, lacunar infarcts, and white matter hyperintensities that can be visualized on MRI is also common. These findings serve to complicate the differential diagnosis among AD, vascular dementia, and mixed states. Functional positron emission tomography (PET) and single photon emission computed tomography (SPECT) have demonstrated consistent patterns of asymmetric parietal and temporal lobe hypometabolism in AD. Despite these findings, current clinical guidelines do not recommend the routine use of PET or SPECT scans because of their high cost and their lack of clear diagnostic usefulness. However, advances in functional scanning may well make them the preferred method of diagnosis in the future. Recent studies have isolated new compounds that can bind to β-amyloid or to tangles and plaques so that they can be visualized in the brain without having to conduct a biopsy. These discoveries may enable clinicians to identify and then to quantify plaque and tangle load to diagnose and stage AD even before the clinical symptoms appear.

Neuropsychologic Testing

Because AD affects the hippocampus early on, the first signs of impairment involve memory encoding into long-term memory. As a result, the most sensitive neuropsychologic tests are usually those of verbal learning with delayed recall. In comparison, tests of digit span will usually be normal in early stages because the immediate or working memory remains intact longer. Tests of executive function and verbal fluency are impaired in the early to middle stages of AD, and the deficits in verbal fluency progress to more advanced degrees of aphasia throughout the course of the illness. In the middle to late stages of AD, neuropsychologic testing reveals a profile of global cognitive impairment across a broad spectrum of individual tests.

Genetic Testing

The purpose of genetic testing for AD ideally is to detect the disease or to determine the relative chance of getting the disease before any symptoms appear. After that point, genetic testing could be used to confirm or to rule out a diagnosis. If testing is conducted, informed consent, guaranteed confidentiality, and genetic counseling both before and after results are available are critical. Unfortunately, genetic testing remains controversial because of a number of ethical and practical concerns. Consequently, most clinicians do not recommend its use as part of routine dementia workup.

A review of the genetics of AD points out the many problems. For an individual with early-onset AD before the age of 50 (fewer than 1% of all cases of AD), the most likely genetic cause would be a mutation on the presenilin 1 gene on chromosome 14. However, many possible mutations could occur on the gene, so a given genetic sequence may prove meaningless if it does not match the known abnormal sequences. For early-onset AD between the ages of 50 and 60, which represents fewer than 5% of all cases, genetic testing would have to sequence the genes for presenilins 1 and 2 and for APP on chromosome 21 completely in the search for specific mutations. Such extensive testing would be expensive, and the yield would not be certain. For late-onset AD, the only available genetic testing is for the APOE4 allele. Although such information may improve the diagnostic certainty, the existing tests lack both the sensitivity and specificity to increase the confidence of the diagnosis by more than 5% to 10%. Although this information may be useful in some circumstances, the combination of the history, examination, and neuropsychologic testing may already be sufficient. The ethics of genetic testing are further discussed in Chapter 16.

Biomarkers

A biomarker represents an anatomic or functional product of AD that can be sampled or measured to make a diagnosis. An ideal biomarker would have to be accurate, reliable, easily obtainable, and inexpensive. It would also have to improve the clinician's ability to identify individuals who actually have AD (sensitivity) and to distinguish AD from other diseases (specificity) over the current practice. Because clinical diagnoses currently have a sensitivity between 85% and 90%, improvement is not a pressing need. Instead, the main advantage of a biomarker would be to provide a quicker, if not more certain, diagnosis. Many such tests, including measuring pupillary dilation in response to anticholinergic eyedrops, performing a skin biopsy for amyloid detection, and sampling for dystrophic olfactory epithelial neurites, have appeared and then receded over time. None of these tests met the goals of the ideal biomarker as previously stated. The only biomarkers currently in use include the following:

- β-Amyloid (measured in the cerebrospinal fluid [CSF]);
- Tau protein (measured in the CSF);
- Neural thread protein/AD7C-NTP (measured in the CSF and urine).

A typical pattern seen in the CSF of patients with AD is a reduced level of 42-amino-acid β-amyloid and an increase in tau protein. The information is limited, however, by the fact that this pattern is also encountered in other conditions. In addition, obtaining a CSF sample requires an invasive spinal tap because data to support the use of blood or urine tests for β-amyloid and tau protein levels are lacking. An even less specific test measures the urine or CSF levels of AD7C-NTP, a protein found in the long axonal processes of neurons and associated with neurofibrillary tangles. The speculation is that this protein may increase in AD and other conditions because it is involved in neuronal repair.

Electroencephalography

Electroencephalography is not commonly used to make a diagnosis of AD, but it may be recommended when delirium is strongly suspected in the differential diagnosis. Characteristic findings include slower background alpha activity (8 Hz) that continues to slow and then disorganizes as the disease progresses. The increased presence of theta and delta activity is also observed.

Treatment of Alzheimer Disease

Essential Concepts

- Factors under study that may reduce the risk of Alzheimer disease (AD) include estrogen replacement therapy, the use of nonsteroidal antiinflammatory drugs (NSAIDs), the intake of antioxidants, B vitamins, statins, and *Ginkgo biloba*.

- No cure is available for AD, but the acetyl-cholinesterase (AChE) inhibitors have proven efficacy in stabilizing its symptoms, including impaired cognition, function, and behavior.

- The AChE inhibitors currently used to treat AD are tacrine, donepezil, rivastigmine, and galantamine.

- The N-methyl-D-aspartate (NMDA)-receptor antagonist memantine has demonstrated an efficacy in treating AD that is similar to the AChE inhibitors.

Although AD remains an incurable disorder, it is not untreatable. Ideally, clinicians would like to prevent the disease from developing, but identifying individuals with the disease before clinical symptoms appear is not yet possible. However, some individuals with a higher risk of AD can be identified (see Table 6.3), and research has identified a number of factors that can reduce their risk. At this time, instead of preventing the disease, the goal is to treat it once it manifests. Several United States Food and Drug Administration (FDA)–approved acetylcholinesterase inhibitors that are currently available stabilize and improve the symptoms, leading to an overall improvement in the course of the disease. This chapter reviews these agents, provides some practical tips on using them, and discusses other compounds and strategies that are either being developed or are being tested to treat and perhaps even to cure AD.

PREVENTIVE AND PROTECTIVE STRATEGIES FOR ALZHEIMER DISEASE

Just as certain factors increase the risk of developing AD, other factors may either reduce that risk or serve a neuroprotective role in blunting the course of the disease. Lifestyle factors that reduce one's risk include involvement in social, physical, and intellectual activities, including higher education earlier in life. A more active lifestyle may possibly help to "exercise" the brain to maximize its function, thus building up a protective cognitive reserve, as Chapter 6 discusses. The prevention of cerebrovascular injury may also reduce the risk of getting AD or prevent a much worse course. This can be accomplished in part through the management of vascular risk factors, such as high blood pressure, elevated cholesterol and lipid levels, diabetes, and tobacco use. Statin medications can lower an individual's cholesterol levels, and they may also have antiinflammatory properties and the ability to block the damaging effects of β-amyloid. Elevated levels of the amino acid homocysteine have been linked to a fivefold increase in the risk of heart attack and stroke and more recently to a threefold increase in the risk of AD. These levels may be reduced by increasing the intake of folate and B vitamins through diet or supplements. The effects of tobacco use are controversial; although smoking increases the risk of cerebrovascular disease, it also provides nicotine, which has a positive effect on cholinergic transmission in the brain. Numerous studies have shown that both rodents and humans tend to perform better on discrete cognitive tests when they are under the influence of nicotine. However, despite the fact that several European studies have shown an inverse relationship between smoking and rates of AD, further research has not confirmed these findings.

Several other common strategies that have been studied for their ability either to prevent or at least to modify the course of AD include the use of antioxidants, antiinflammatory agents, estrogen, and *Ginkgo biloba*. Each strategy is reviewed in this chapter, with practical tips on its use.

Antioxidant Therapy

As Chapter 6 describes, one proposal implicates an oxidative mechanism as possibly being partially responsible for age-related neuronal degeneration, perhaps contributing to the development of AD. In the brain of an individual with AD, β-amyloid can generate cytotoxic hydrogen peroxide and other free radicals. One theory suggests that *vitamin E* (α-tocopherol), a potent antioxidant, may have a neuroprotective role by blunting free radical damage to the brain. In one study, 341 patients with moderately severe AD received either 2,000 IU vitamin E per day (1,000 IU twice daily), 10 mg of selegiline daily, both, or a placebo for 2 years. Measured end points included the loss of activities of daily living, more severe dementia, long-term care placement, and death. Both vitamin E and selegiline slowed the progression of AD to several end points, and the use of each agent alone produced better results than did their combination. No benefit on cognitive measures was found with either agent.

Clearly, no evidence as yet suggests that vitamin E prevents AD or that it significantly slows the disease progression; the only evidence that exists suggests that high-dose vitamin E may yield mild functional improvement. Most individuals taking a multivitamin receive within the recommended daily allowance (RDA) for vitamin E of 15 to 45 IU, whereas individuals on actual supplements may be receiving 200 to 800 IU daily. The study, however, used doses that were five to 10 times greater. Such a high dose may be necessary due to vitamin E's low penetration of the central nervous system. Vitamin E tends to be well tolerated, even at high doses, although the potential side effects include nausea, diarrhea, fatigue, muscle weakness, and bruising. Bleeding becomes more of a concern when vitamin E is combined with anticoagulants.

Selegiline (Eldepryl, L-deprenyl) increases catecholamines in the brain by selectively inhibiting the metabolic enzyme monoamine oxidase B (MAO-B). In this capacity, it has been used as an antidepressant agent (to boost levels of norepinephrine) and a treatment for Parkinson disease (to boost levels of dopamine). In AD, MAO-B activity increases significantly, which could possibly lead to the enhanced oxidative deamination of monoamines. The resultant increase in free radicals may increase the neuronal damage. Similar to vitamin E, selegiline may be neuroprotective because of its antioxidant properties, and, in the study cited previously, it was shown to decrease the rate of functional decline in AD and to delay nursing home placement. The main limitation of selegiline is its side effect profile. MAO inhibitors have numerous side effects, including nausea, weight gain, and orthostasis. In addition, MAO inhibitors can trigger a potentially deadly hypertensive crisis when they are combined with foods that contain tyramine (e.g., aged cheese, wine) and with certain medications, such as selective serotonin reuptake inhibitor antidepressants and sympathomimetic agents. Selegiline can also be quite activating for some individuals because amphetamine is one of its metabolites. By virtue of being a selective MAO-B inhibitor, selegiline has a safer profile than do the nonselective MAO inhibitors, and it can be used in doses as high as 10 mg without the need to implement a restrictive diet and without a high risk of a hypertensive crisis. This window of safety is helpful because the typical daily dose for an older individual is 5 to 10 mg per day. Unfortunately, the potential benefit from selegiline is modest at best, and, even at the lower doses, most physicians and many pharmacists worry about the remote possibility of a hypertensive crisis. In practice, selegiline is neither recommended nor widely accepted as a treatment for AD.

Antiinflammatory Medications

Substantial evidence shows that an inflammatory process triggered by the presence of β-amyloid and mediated by the immune system plays a key role in the pathogenesis of AD. The logical conclusion, then, is that antiinflammatory agents would reduce the risk of developing AD or that they might serve to ameliorate the damage caused by inflammation. In fact, researchers have hypothesized that the lower rates of AD in individuals with rheumatoid arthritis are the direct result of their long-term NSAID use. In a longitudinal study of NSAIDs (mainly ibuprofen), aspirin, and acetaminophen taken for at least 2 years, the relative risk of AD decreased with increasing duration of NSAID use but not with use of aspirin or acetaminophen. Other studies have found benefit with the use of indomethacin and more recently with aspirin. Cyclooxygenase-2 inhibitors, such as celecoxib (Celebrex) and rofecoxib (Vioxx), have yet to demonstrate results comparable to those seen with ibuprofen. More recent prospective research has called into question the actual preventive or protective role of NSAIDs with respect to AD. In addition, the risk of gastritis and other serious side effects from long-term use might well outweigh its benefits. No verdict has been made on whether NSAIDs should be used, and they are not currently recommended for AD prevention.

Estrogen

Many reasons exist for why estrogen may play a role in reducing the risk of AD. The possible roles of estrogen include promoting neural growth and synapse formation, facilitating memory formation, and increasing cerebral blood flow, and it may even have antioxidant properties. Not surprisingly, estrogen receptors are found in brain areas related to cognition. Several studies have demonstrated an inverse relationship between postmenopausal hormone replacement therapy (HRT) and the relative risk of developing AD. A metaanalysis that reviewed cumulative data from 10 studies suggested a 29% risk reduction with the use of HRT. Another study of 472 women on HRT found a 54% reduction in the risk of developing AD. More recent research has cast doubt on the benefits of HRT, and it has even suggested an *increased* risk of HRT with certain HRT combinations. Because men obviously are not ideal candidates for estrogen, ongoing research is trying to determine whether testosterone serves a protective role for men.

Given this evidence, estrogen use has not been routinely promoted as a preventive treatment of AD in women. Similar to NSAID use, the potential benefits of estrogen for AD have to be weighed against the potential side effects, including an increased risk of ovarian and breast cancer. Many women are simply not good candidates for HRT for a variety of reasons, and other women are becoming increasingly concerned by the potential cancer risk and growing skepticism over the previously reported benefits for postmenopausal women.

Ginkgo biloba

In Chinese medicine, extracts from leaves of the *Ginkgo biloba* tree have been used for thousands of years for their hypothesized benefits on brain function. Modern-day research has suggested that *Ginkgo biloba* extracts may have both antioxidant and antiinflammatory properties and that they may increase cerebral circulation. In a 52-week, randomized, double-blind, placebo-controlled study of *Ginkgo biloba* in patients with mild to moderate dementia, subjects taking 40 mg of *Ginkgo biloba* three times daily demonstrated an extremely small, but statistically significant, difference on a measure of cognitive function compared with the placebo group. *Ginkgo biloba* was well tolerated compared with the placebo. However, more extensive data supporting the benefits of *Ginkgo biloba* in AD do not exist, despite the fact that many individuals take it. The ongoing clinical trials of *Ginkgo biloba* should help to clarify this. At the present time, most memory disorder centers do not routinely prescribe *Ginkgo biloba* extract. Although many people assume that it is safe because it is labeled a "natural herbal extract," *Ginkgo biloba* has been associated with clotting disturbances and adverse interactions with anesthesia.

Ergoloid Mesylates

Ergoloid mesylates (Hydergine [Novartis, East Hanover, New Jersey]) consist of several hydrogenated alkaloids of ergot (a rye fungus), and they were a popular treatment of dementia in the 1970s. It remains a popular treatment of dementia in Europe, where it is sold with a similar ergot derivative called nicergoline (Sermion). Although its mechanism of action has never been clarified, it is thought to work as a cerebral vasodilator, and it may also have antioxidant properties.

Ergoloid mesylates have been studied in numerous clinical trials, including seven that were double blind and placebo controlled. The latter trials have demonstrated some degree of improvement in at least 50% of subjects. In patients with AD, the cognitive and behavioral effects of ergoloid mesylates were relatively mild. In vascular dementia, both cognition and behavior showed modest improvement. Although one critical review of ergoloid mesylates studies highlights the supportive data, it also notes that much of the research to date has consisted of small samples without consistent methods of diagnosis. The efficacy of ergoloid mesylates has also been called into question, which may account for the significant decline in its use, especially since the advent of the AChE inhibitors.

The doses range from 1.5 to 12 mg per day, although the most typical dose is 3 to 6 mg per day, divided into three doses (1 to 2 mg three times daily). It is also sold in 4.5-mg tablets and as an oral solution. Ergoloid mesylates have a relatively safe side effect profile, even with long-term use; the most common side effects include mild nausea or other gastrointestinal distress and headache.

TREATMENT OF ALZHEIMER DISEASE: BEYOND PREVENTION AND PROTECTION

The treatment strategies reviewed thus far have been aimed at reducing the risk of developing AD more than treating the disease itself. However, none has become standard care for AD because of either controversial findings or potential side effects. Treatments that are currently being studied or used to treat AD attempt to block either the disease process itself or the neuronal injury as a result of this process. Based on the current understanding of AD pathology, the following strategies lay the foundation for potential treatments.

Prevent or Decrease the Production of Amyloid Precursor Protein

Because amyloid precursor protein (APP) is a normal protein found in neurons, preventing or decreasing its production might be hazardous. The key may lie in preventing it from being overexpressed, as may happen during the pathologic process of AD, perhaps as part of an inflammatory response.

Inhibit the Formation and/or the Effects of β-Amyloid

Because β-amyloid is believed to be the central "culprit" in AD, several approaches to treatment may exist. These include the following: inhibiting its formation from APP, preventing the formation of insoluble β-pleated sheets of β-amyloid, blocking its damaging effects, or causing its breakdown once it forms. Ongoing research has been focusing on pharmaceutical agents that act as *secretase inhibitors* to prevent the conversion of APP to β-amyloid. Several candidate compounds are being investigated. Such agents could ostensibly arrest or even cure AD, assuming, of course, that amyloid is the actual cause.

Attempts have also been made to develop a *vaccine* to counteract β-amyloid. A clinical trial of a vaccine composed of amyloid protein fragments generated much excitement due to earlier studies with transgenic mice that showed that it prevented amyloid plaque formation and led to the dissolution of formed plaque. Clinical trials in humans, however, had to be discontinued because of the occurrence of encephalitis in several subjects. Despite this setback, evidence indicates that the vaccine may have reduced plaques in several subjects. The search for a safer vaccine continues along several fronts.

Neotrofin (leteprinim potassium) is an agent that increases neural growth factor; it has been demonstrated to decrease the levels of β-amyloid in cell cultures. Preliminary clinical trials with patients with AD found improvement on both the cognitive subscale of the Alzheimer's Disease Assessment Scale (ADAS-Cog) and a global change rating scale; however, the improvement was not to a level of statistical significance over the placebo. A newer strategy to treat AD has isolated a protein called *SAP* that blocks the degradation of amyloid; inhibition of this protein may theoretically help to remove β-amyloid from the brain.

Prevent Destabilization of Tau Protein

The role of amyloid versus tau protein in the pathogenesis of AD is still being debated, but neurofibrillary tangles remain a pathologic hallmark. Researchers are trying to identify ways to prevent the hyperphosphorylization and subsequent destabilization of the tau protein.

Other Strategies

Other categories of medications used to treat AD have included the following:

- NMDA receptor antagonists;
- Neural growth factors;
- Serotonergic and dopaminergic agents;
- Chelating agents (aluminum, copper, and iron);
- Neuronal membrane stabilizers.

Memantine is a new type of AD medication that blocks glutamate or NMDA receptor excitotoxicity, leading to less neuronal injury in AD. Research has demonstrated its efficacy in patients with AD with moderate to severe symptoms in terms of both cognition and function. Memantine is widely used in Europe, and it is expected to receive FDA approval to be sold in the United States. Memantine is typically titrated in 5-mg increments to a total dose of 10 mg twice daily. Although dozens of other compounds have been tested in patients with AD, beyond those that have been mentioned here, few have moved beyond preliminary research or have demonstrated significant efficacy in AD. Chelating agents, in particular, were studied in response to concerns that the accumulation of metals, such as aluminum, in the brain may cause AD. However, extensive research on aluminum and other metals has been unrevealing. Instead, the standard treatment for AD since 1989 has been based on the use of the AChE inhibitors.

Enhance Cholinergic Function

As Chapter 6 describes, the cholinergic hypothesis posits that a deficiency of acetylcholine (ACh) in the brain is primarily responsible for the cognitive impairment seen in AD. Approximately 40 years ago, researchers first recognized that a reduction of cholinergic function occurs in the brains of those with AD. What began as an observation on the deficiencies of choline acetyltransferase in postmortem brain samples grew into the realization that the cholinergic cell bodies were destroyed by the disease process.

In fact, concentration of ACh is reduced by 90% in the brains of those with AD. Further proof for the cholinergic hypothesis lies in the fact that cognitive impairment induced by intravenous anticholinergic agents can be reversed by cholinergic antidotes. The goal of treatment, then, is to improve cognitive deficits in AD by increasing the levels of ACh in the brain. The following three potential strategies could be used to accomplish this: (a) increase synthesis and release of ACh, (b) block ACh degradation by inhibiting the enzyme AChE, and (c) increase cholinergic transmission with cholinergic receptor agonists that activate either muscarinic or nicotinic receptors.

The first strategy that researchers devised was the intravenous administration of the AChE inhibitor *physostigmine* (Antilirium) to increase ACh by inhibiting its metabolism. Studies indicated that this therapy did lead to some improvement on cognitive tests and that it could reverse the cognitive effects of anticholinergic agents, such as scopolamine; however, it had no clear effects on the progression of AD. Even if physostigmine can treat AD, its use is impractical given its extremely short half-life (20 to 120 minutes), the need for intravenous administration, and the prominent cholinergic side effects (e.g., nausea, vomiting, diarrhea, sweating, flushing, bradycardia). A longer acting form of physostigmine is now being studied. Aside from its use in AD, physostigmine is used clinically to reverse drug-induced anticholinergic delirium.

Other strategies have used ACh precursors such as *lecithin* (phosphatidylcholine) and *choline*, both of which are widely available in health food stores. However, the oral use of these precursors was not found to benefit individuals with AD. In addition, lecithin has one particularly bothersome side effect— because it is derived from fish oil, individuals who take large doses may emit a fishy odor. Some ongoing research is looking at *acetyl-L-carnitine*, a protein found in mitochondria that is involved in the synthesis and release of ACh. Acetyl-L-carnitine has shown some benefit over a placebo in a double-blind, placebo-controlled study of 130 individuals with AD. However, more data are needed to support it use as an effective treatment.

Inhibit Acetylcholinesterase

The fact that, despite a wealth of data on the AChE inhibitors, they do not cure AD must be emphasized at the start. Their benefits, although modest at best, can, however, have important effects on the lives and the overall care of individuals with AD. Studies have consistently shown the following benefits for all of the AChE inhibitors:

- Improvement and/or stabilization of cognition for 10 to 12 months, followed by a long-term decrease in the degree of decline compared with the placebo;
- Improvement and/or stabilization in functional abilities;
- Overall (global) improvement over the placebo;
- Stabilization in the prevalence of behavioral problems;
- Delayed nursing home placement;
- Decreased caregiver stress and burden;
- Increased caregiver respite time;
- Overall cost savings.

All AChE inhibitors currently on the market are believed to work by increasing the levels of ACh in the brain. Rivastigmine also inhibits the related enzyme butyrylcholinesterase that may be more prevalent in the later stages of the disease. Galantamine also serves as an allosteric modulator of the presynaptic nicotinic receptors, which are associated with the enhanced release of ACh. The AChE inhibitors that are currently available are listed in Table 7.1, with several of their important characteristics.

Because AChE inhibitors can increase ACh levels in the periphery, the potential side effects include the increased secretion of gastric acid, increased bronchial secretions, vagotonic effects on the heart that can exacerbate bradyarrhyth-

TABLE 7.1. Acetylcholinesterase Inhibitors

Drug (brand name)	Dosing guidelines
Tacrine (Cognex) (10-mg, 20-mg, 30-mg, 40-mg capsules)	Start at 10 mg p.o. q.i.d. Titrate every 4 wk by 40 mg to maximum of 40 mg q.i.d. Check LFTs every 2 wk for 16 wk, then every 3 mo.
Donepezil (Aricept) (5-mg, 10-mg tablets)	Start at 5 mg p.o. q.h.s. Titrate after 4 wk to 10 mg p.o. q.h.s. Maximal daily dose of 15 mg.
Rivastigmine (Exelon) (1.5-mg, 3-mg, 4.5-mg, 6-mg capsules and oral solution)	Start at 1.5 mg p.o. b.i.d. with meals. Titrate every 2–4 wk by 1.5–3 mg/wk to dose of 3–6 mg p.o. b.i.d.
Galantamine (Reminyl) (4-mg, 8-mg, 12-mg tablets and oral solution)	Start at 4 mg p.o. b.i.d. with meals. Titrate after 4 wk to 8 mg p.o. b.i.d. Maximal daily dose of 24 mg.

Abbreviations: b.i.d., twice daily; LFTs, liver function tests; p.o., by mouth; q.h.s., every night; q.i.d., four times daily.

mias, and the potentiation of the effects of succinylcholine in anesthesia. The most common are usually the gastrointestinal-related side effects, including nausea, vomiting, anorexia, and diarrhea. Slow titration and administration with food can decrease the frequency and severity of these effects. Even when they do occur, the side effects tend to abate after several days as the individual's tolerance builds, or they may be relieved by temporary dose reduction. However, the initiation of treatment should be avoided in an individual with active peptic ulcer disease, unstable bradycardia, acute pulmonary disease, or congestive heart failure. AChE inhibitor treatment may be appropriate when the latter medical conditions have been stabilized.

The FDA required the clinical trials of the AChE inhibitors to measure the subjects' cognitive performance on the ADAS-Cog and the Global Evaluation Scale (GES), a scale rating global improvement. The ADAS-Cog is an 11-item, 70-point scale that assesses domains of memory, orientation, language, and daily function. A typical individual with AD may increase 7 to 10 points per year on the scale. Clinically significant improvement is indicated by a drop of at least 4 points. Studies for AChE inhibitors have also looked at measures of function, behavior, and caregiver burden. The typical course of individuals on AChE inhibitors versus those on a placebo is demonstrated graphically in Fig. 7.1, which also illustrates the course alteration in AD when the patient is put on active medication at a later time. This graph represents consistent findings across *all* studies with *all* the AChE inhibitors currently on the market. In general, AChE inhibitors improve or stabilize symptoms above or at baseline in the average patient for 10 to 12 months, after which a slow, but steady, decline continues in a manner parallel to, but always better than, the average individual not on treatment. Individuals on placebo who are later put on an AChE inhibitor improve, but they never achieve the level of those started earlier. When the AChE inhibitor is stopped, the levels of performance quickly decline, and they approximate those of individuals without previous treatment. In essence, those cognitive skills lost in AD are never regained, thus constituting an argument for early and consistent use of AChE inhibitors. The clinician must keep this graph in mind when he or she is treating a patient and is wondering about the potential benefits if they are not immediately discernible.

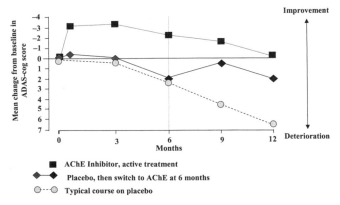

FIG. 7.1. The typical effects of acetylcholinesterase (AChE) inhibitors on cognition in patients with Alzheimer disease. The change in scores on the cognitive subscale of the Alzheimer's Disease Assessment Scale for a double-blind, placebo-controlled, 6-month trial, followed by an open-label, 6-month extension trial of an AChE inhibitor. (From Raskind MA, Peskind ER, Wessel T, Yuan W. Galantamine in AD: a 6-month randomized, placebo-controlled trial with a 6-month extension. *Neurology* 2000;54:2261–2268, with permission.)

KEY POINT

When treating someone with an AChE inhibitor, avoid expectations for a cure or even of a dramatic change in the rate of decline. Such expectations are certain to leave you disappointed, perhaps leading you to withdraw the treatment prematurely. Consider the following analogy: your patient is sitting in a boat with a hole in the bottom, slowly sinking. You do not have a way to plug the hole to stop the water from coming in (i.e., there is no cure), but you can bail out water to keep him or her afloat for a longer period. In essence, this is what you are doing for your patient—keeping his or her cognitive abilities "afloat" longer than if he or she were not on any medication.

Tacrine (Cognex) is a reversible AChE inhibitor, and it was the first one on the market in 1992. Clinical trials in individuals with mild to moderate AD found that those on tacrine performed significantly better than those receiving the placebo on the ADAS-Cog and the GES. Dosing starts at 10 mg orally four times daily (40 mg per day) with titration every 4 to 6 weeks to 80, 120, and then 160 mg orally per day in four doses. The common side effects include nausea, vomiting, diarrhea, dyspepsia, headache, and myalgias. Tacrine is no longer widely used because nearly 50% of individuals on the medication experience liver transaminase elevations, a problem not encountered with the newer AChE inhibitors.

Donepezil (Aricept), the second reversible cholinesterase inhibitor that came on the market, was found, like tacrine, to be superior to the placebo on the ADAS-Cog and the GES. The data indicated that 82% of the treated patients experienced either improvement in cognition or no decline. More recent data have demonstrated the stabilization of both daily function and behavioral problems. Long-term studies of patients on donepezil indicate that, although the symptoms of AD continue to progress, the curve of the decline is always better on active medication. In general, donepezil is well tolerated, and its most common side effects include nausea, vomiting, diarrhea, headache, insomnia, vivid dreams, and dizziness. With a half-life of 70 hours, donepezil can be dosed once daily, starting at 5 mg orally per day and increasing to 10 mg per day, if tolerated, after 4 to 6 weeks. Some clinicians push the dose as high as 15 mg orally per day. Donepezil has no significant effects on liver function and no significant drug–drug interactions.

Rivastigmine (Exelon), the third AChE inhibitor on the market, is a reversible AChE and butyrylcholinesterase inhibitor. Like its predecessors, it was found in clinical trials to be superior to the placebo on both the ADAS-Cog and the GES. In addition, clinical trials with rivastigmine have demonstrated the stabilization of daily function and behavioral problems. Patients with moderately severe symptoms of AD also show benefit in terms of both cognition and behavior. Recent studies found benefit in patients with both AD and vascular risk factors and in patients with dementia with Lewy bodies. Rivastigmine has a short half-life of 1.5 hours but a 10-hour duration of cholinesterase inhibition. Dosing starts at 1.5 mg orally twice daily and increases every 3 to 4 weeks to 3, 4.5, and 6 mg twice daily, as tolerated. In clinical trials involving a relatively rigorous titration schedule, rivastigmine was associated with significant gastrointestinal effects, including nausea, vomiting, anorexia, and weight loss. These tend to be the most frequent side effects, although the risk of these can be minimized with slow titration and administration with meals. Furthermore, the side effects do become less frequent over the course of treatment. Rivastigmine does not have any significant drug–drug interactions.

Galantamine (Reminyl) was the fourth reversible AChE inhibitor on the market. It has a dual mechanism of action, serving as an AChE inhibitor and potentially increasing cholinergic activity by activating presynaptic nicotinic receptors. Like all other AChE inhibitors, galantamine was found superior to the placebo in clinical trials using the ADAS-Cog and the GES. In addition, galantamine has been found to stabilize both function and behavioral problems, to improve caregiver stress, and to increase the caregiver's respite time. Research has also found that galantamine is beneficial for both AD with vascular risk factors and vascular dementia itself. Galantamine is administered with meals starting at 4 mg orally twice daily and is then increased to 8 mg orally twice daily after 4 weeks. The clinician does have the option of going to 12 mg orally twice daily; individuals in clinical trials who were on the 24-mg daily dose did numerically better on tests, although the difference was not statistically significant. These findings suggest at least the possibility that the higher dose may bring additional benefits to some patients. The side effects are usually gastrointestinal related, as with the other AChE inhibitors. Ketoconazole, erythromycin, and paroxetine are concomitant medications that may potentially increase the levels of galantamine, although a dose reduction of galantamine is not always necessary; instead, closer patient monitoring is warranted.

 TIP

Is one AChE inhibitor better than another? Should I switch?

Research has not conclusively demonstrated that any one AChE inhibitor is superior to another. No clear basis, then, exists to recommend automatically switching someone from one AChE inhibitor to another to improve symptoms. However, if you do decide to switch for reasons of efficacy, make sure that you have pushed the first agent to the maximal recommended dose. If you still plan to change, a clean switch can be made by stopping the existing agent on day 1 and starting the new agent at its starting dose on day 2. If you are switching because of side effects, stop the original agent and allow the side effects to subside before starting the new agent.

OTHER CHOLINERGIC AGENTS

Several new AChE inhibitors are being studied, although two—*velnacrine* and *eptastigmine*—have been associated with significant side effects that may preclude their coming on the market. *Metrifonate* is an organophosphate agent that binds to AChE to provide a gradual, dose-dependent cholinomimetic effect through long-lasting inhibition. Despite being a well-studied medication with good efficacy for AD symptoms, metrifonate was pulled from the process of obtaining FDA approval because of severe side effects. Two medications that enhance cholinergic function by directly activating the muscarinic subtype of ACh receptors, *xanomeline* and *oxotremorine*, have demonstrated some improvement in patients with AD but with less consistency than the AChE inhibitors and with significant side effects.

8   Vascular Dementia

Essential Concepts

- Vascular dementia (VaD) is the second most common form of dementia. VaD is caused by brain damage due to strokes.
- Cortical VaD usually results from large cerebral vessel strokes. The symptoms vary depending on the location of the stroke.
- Subcortical VaD commonly results from small lacunar infarcts. Its symptoms include frontal lobe impairment due to damage to the frontal and/or subcortical neural circuits.
- Treatment of VaD involves reducing the risk factors for stroke and boosting cholinergic function with acetylcholinesterase inhibitors.

VaD, previously known as *multiinfarct dementia*, is the second most common form of dementia after Alzheimer disease (AD), affecting as many as 25% of individuals with dementia. VaD may resemble AD clinically, but its etiology is distinct. It is caused by focal or diffuse cortical or subcortical brain damage as a result of cerebrovascular disease. Secondary causes of VaD are embolic strokes resulting from cardiovascular events (i.e., emboli generated during arrhythmias, such as atrial fibrillation) or from carotid artery atheromatous plaques. Given this etiology, the presence of vascular lesions on brain scans represents a key diagnostic feature of VaD. The prevalence rates for VaD are tied into the rates of stroke; as a result, the rate of VaD increases nearly 200-fold from the age of 60 years to that of 90, but this includes a significant overlap with AD. Those individuals with the greatest risk of VaD are those at risk for stroke, including a history of atherosclerosis, hypertension, hyperlipidemia, arrhythmias, diabetes mellitus, and tobacco use. Not surprisingly, the prevalence rates of VaD have declined as a result of improvements in stroke prevention and treatment.

CLINICAL VIGNETTE

Mr. Anthony was a 75-year-old advertising executive with diabetes, coronary heart disease, and hypertension who enjoyed smoking cigars. During a ski trip in Utah, he had a stroke that resulted in right-sided hemiparesis and mild aphasia. With aggressive rehabilitation, he was able to walk with a cane and to communicate with only a mild degree of word-finding difficulty. However, 4 months after the stroke, his wife reported that his short-term memory was poor and that he was prone to fits of anger. Six months after his stroke, Mr. Anthony was forced to retire because he was unable to manage his accounts. Treatment for depression reduced his irritability, but the cognitive impairment persisted. Mr. Anthony was able to control his diet and blood pressure, but he continued to smoke. Two years after his stroke, he had another one that left him severely aphasic and unable to walk. Physical and occupational therapy led to moderate physical improvement, but his cognition remained poor.

DIAGNOSTIC CRITERIA

The following two sets of diagnostic criteria are commonly used for VaD: the *Diagnostic and Statistical Manual of Mental Disorders*, Fourth Edition, Text Revision criteria and the National Institute of Neurological Disorders and Stroke–Association Internationale pour la Recherche et l'Enseignement en Neurosciences (NINDS–AIREN) criteria. These are listed in Tables 8.1 and 8.2, respectively. Both sets focus on the relationship between the presence of cerebrovascular disease or the occurrence of strokes and the onset of dementia symptoms. The NINDS–AIREN criteria also account for the probability of the diagnosis.

RELEVANCE OF STROKE

Each year an estimated 500,000 to 700,000 individuals in the United States have strokes. Of this number, researchers have found that, after 3 months, approximately 25% to 30% of these individuals develop dementia, representing 125,000

TABLE 8.1. *Diagnostic and Statistical Manual of Mental Disorders*, Fourth Edition, Text Revision, Criteria for Vascular Dementia

---

A. The development of multiple cognitive deficits manifested by both memory impairment and one or more of the following: aphasia, apraxia, agnosia, and disturbances in executive functioning

B. The cognitive deficits represent a decline from previous functioning and cause significant impairment in social or occupational functioning

C. Focal neurologic signs and symptoms or other evidence of cerebrovascular disease is judged to be etiologically related to the disturbance

D. The deficits do not occur exclusively during the course of a delirium

---

From American Psychiatric Association. *Diagnostic and statistical manual of mental disorders,* fourth edition, text revision. Washington, D.C.: American Psychiatric Association, 2000, with permission.

new cases of VaD per year, compared with nearly 360,000 cases of AD. Four types of cerebrovascular accident or stroke can occur, and all are associated with VaD. These include the following:

1. **Thrombotic:** This is the most common form of stroke; tissue infarct or death occurs due to thrombosis or blockage of an artery in the brain that is caused by the buildup of atheromatous plaque.

2. **Embolic:** Damage to brain tissue results from arterial blockage by a fragment or emboli of atheromatous material or a blood clot from either the carotid arteries or the heart. Embolic events account for one-third of all strokes.

3. **Lacunar:** These are small strokes, sometimes lacking overt clinical symptoms, that result from the occlusion of small penetrating cerebral arteries in the deeper, noncortical regions of the brain. They represent one-fifth of all strokes.

4. **Hemorrhagic:** This is the most serious, but least common, type of stroke that causes brain damage due to bleeding in the brain, usually as a result of ruptured aneurysms or arteriovenous malformations. They are commonly associated with high blood pressure or anticoagulation therapy.

Regardless of the type of stroke, the results of any given stroke are unpredictable. However, the likelihood of dementia increases significantly with left-sided lesions; tissue death

TABLE 8.2. National Institute of Neurological Disorders and Stroke–Association International pour la Recherche et l'Enseignementen Neurosciences Diagnostic Criteria for the Diagnosis of Vascular Dementia

Probable vascular dementia
Dementia defined by impairment of memory and two or more of the following: orientation, attention, language, visuospatial functions, executive function, motor control, and praxis
Evidence of CVD, such as focal neurologic symptoms or findings on neuroimaging
Relationship between dementia and CVD likely given either the onset of dementia within 3 months after stroke or abrupt cognitive deterioration or a stepwise progression of cognitive deficits
Clinical features include (a) gait disturbances and falls, (b) urinary symptoms not explained by urologic disease, (c) personality and mood changes, and (d) subcortical symptoms such as psychomotor retardation and abnormal executive function
Definite vascular dementia
Clinical criteria for probable VaD, histopathologic evidence of CVD obtained from biopsy or autopsy, neurofibrillary tangles and presence of neuritic plaques not exceeding those expected for age, and absence of other clinical or pathologic disorder capable of producing dementia
Possible vascular dementia
Dementia (as described above) with focal neurologic signs but without evidence of CVD by neuroimaging or without temporal relationship to stroke or in patients with subtle onset and variable course of cognitive deficits and evidence of relevant CVD
Unlikely vascular dementia
Dementia as described above but with the absence of focal neurologic signs or focal brain lesions on neuroimaging

Abbreviation: CVD, cerebrovascular disease.
Adapted from Roman GC, Tatemichi TK, Erkinjuntti T, et al. Vascular dementia: diagnostic criteria for research studies. Report of the NINDS–AIREN International Workshop. *Neurology* 1993;43:250–260, with permission.

of more than 50 to 100 cm^3; stroke symptoms, such as dysphagia, gait impairment, and urinary incontinence; and stroke complications, including seizures, arrhythmias, pneumonia, and hypotension. Strokes that affect the more influential areas of brain function have a greater likelihood of producing VaD, especially when preexisting damage from prior strokes or other injury is present. In addition, an increased risk of dementia after stroke has been associated with older age, lower education and income levels, tobacco use, a family history of dementia, and a medical history of coronary artery disease and diabetes mellitus.

CLASSIFICATION OF VASCULAR DEMENTIA

VaD can be classified in several ways based on the type, location, and time course of the vascular injury. Classification by types of vascular injury includes the following:

- VaD due to large vessel disease: the stroke affects a large tissue area, such as in the distribution of anterior, posterior, or middle cerebral arteries;
- VaD due to small vessel disease: smaller strokes, especially lacunae, that result in accumulating damage.

In one review, half of all cases of VaD were due to small vessel disease, one-fourth of the cases were due to large vessel lesions in both the cortical and subcortical areas, and the remainder included elements of both. The most common artery that is affected is the middle cerebral.

The classification by location of vascular injury includes *cortical* VaD and *subcortical* VaD. Cortical damage is usually associated with thrombosis and less so with embolic or hemorrhagic events. Less common, non–cerebrovascular accidents that can cause cortical damage include venous thrombosis, hypoperfusion, trauma, and diffuse microinfarcts. Subcortical VaD is usually associated with the presence of multiple lacunar infarcts in the region of the basal ganglia, thalamus, pons, and surrounding white matter tracts. This variant is sometimes referred to as simply a *lacunar state*. Other major forms of subcortical VaD include the following:

> *Binswanger disease,* also known as subcortical arteriosclerotic encephalopathy or ischemic periventricular leukoencephalopathy, is a slowly progressive dementia associated with chronic hypertension. It is characterized by damage to small, penetrating blood vessels in subcortical regions that results in episodic hypoperfusion and white matter degeneration.
>
> *Cerebral autosomal dominant arteriopathy with subcortical infarcts and leukoencephalopathy* (CADASIL) is an autosomal dominant disorder mapped to chromosome 19

that produces a slowly progressive dementia in adults, usually striking in the mid-40s. It involves a microangiopathic process that affects small arterioles and capillaries, resulting in small ischemic infarcts throughout subcortical structures. CADASIL may progress over 20 years and may involve transient ischemic attacks and strokes, focal neurologic symptoms, headaches, mood disorders, and seizures, in addition to dementia.

Cerebral amyloid angiopathy (CAA) represents a group of disorders characterized by the deposition of β-amyloid pprotein in cerebral blood vessels, resulting in recurrent lobar hemorrhages, ischemic strokes, and evolving dementia. Several different familial forms of CAA exist, and the transmission is autosomal dominant.

A third way to classify VaD is by its time course, *acute* versus *subacute*. Acute-onset VaD occurs after a clinically evident stroke, and it can include both single or recurrent cortical and subcortical events. Subacute VaD usually refers to subcortical syndromes that involve progressive dementia with a fluctuating course and without an obvious temporal relationship to clinical strokes.

CLINICAL SYMPTOMS OF VASCULAR DEMENTIA

Theoretically, the clinical symptoms of VaD should reflect the site(s) of cerebral injury. The complexity of neural connections in the brain, however, often makes actually correlating the symptoms with the anatomic lesions difficult. For clinical diagnosis, then, the most practical distinction that should be made is that between the cortical and subcortical types of VaD.

Cortical VaD primarily involves memory dysfunction and one or more of the following: apraxia, aphasia, agnosia, and executive dysfunction. The associated neurologic impairment is most often characterized by hemiplegia or paresis contralateral to the lesion. The exact form of cognitive impairment due to cortical injury depends first on whether the dominant or nondominant hemisphere is affected (most individuals are left-hemisphere dominant) and then on the particular lobe(s) affected as follows: frontal, parietal, occipital, and temporal. Table 8.3 provides a general guide for correlating the clinical symptoms of cortical impairment with known areas of damage.

TABLE 8.3. Cognitive Effects of Cortical Stroke

Lobe	Focal neurologic and cognitive symptoms
Frontal	Impaired executive functioning
	Impaired immediate memory
	Slowed cognitive processing and activity, poor concentration
	Impairments in judgment, insight, and behavioral control
	Personality changes: apathy or inappropriate and disinhibited behaviors
	Perseveration of words, sounds, or behaviors
	Disinhibited reflexes and/or frontal release signs
	Contralateral hemiplegia or paresis
	Broca aphasia (nonfluent) from a lesion on the dominant side
	Dysprosody (impaired inflection of speech) from lesion on the nondominant side
	Impaired coordination of ocular movements
	Pseudobulbar palsy (emotional incontinence) due to bilateral lesions
	Dorsolateral prefrontal lesions lead to impairment in executive dysfunction
	Orbitofrontal lesions lead to disinhibition, lability, impulsivity, anosmia, distractibility, and perseveration
	Mediofrontal and/or anterior cingulate lesions lead to apathy, personality flattening, akinetic mutism, and impaired task follow-through
Occipital	Visual agnosias for objects, colors, and faces (prosopagnosia)
	Reading impairment and/or dyslexia
	Panoramic visual impairment
	Visual field cuts (homonymous hemianopsia)
	Visual illusions and hallucinations (often of shapes, colors)
	Visual auras associated with occipital seizures
	Alexia without agraphia (lesion on the dominant side and adjacent corpus callosum)
	Balint syndrome (visual inattention and poor tracking due to bilateral lesions)
	Anton syndrome (visual anosognosia, denial of blindness)
	Cortical blindness

TABLE 8.3. *Continued.*

Lobe	Focal neurologic and cognitive symptoms
Parietal	Cortical sensory impairment (hemianesthesia with large lesions)
	Mild hemiparesis
	Visual field cuts (homonymous hemianopsia)
Dominant side	Agraphia (impaired writing ability)
	Acalculia (impaired mathematical ability)
	Reading impairment and/or dyslexia
	Right–left confusion
	Aphasia (fluent)
	Apraxias (ideomotor, simple tasks; ideational, complex tasks)
	Astereognosia (impaired tactile recognition of objects)
	Gerstmann syndrome (agraphia, left–right confusion, finger agnosia, alexia, and acalculia due to a lesion in the dominant posterior parietal and/or angular gyrus)
Nondominant side	Visuospatial and visuoconstructional impairment and apraxias
	Dressing apraxia
	Neglect of dominant side (autotopagnosia)
	Neglect or denial of illness (anosognosia)
Temporal	Impaired memory processing (hippocampus, medial temporal lobe)
	Impaired cortical hearing (lesions in Heschl gyrus)
	Hallucinations (in all sensory modalities)
	Changes in emotional and behavioral expression (with limbic involvement)
	Klüver–Bucy syndrome (apathy, placidity, oral exploratory behaviors, hypersexuality, hyperphagia) due to bilateral lesions
	Visual field cuts (homonymous upper quadrantanopia)
Dominant side	Wernicke aphasia (fluent)
	Amusia (impaired musical appreciation)
Nondominant side	Sound agnosia
	Dysprosody (impaired production and interpretation of speech inflection)

From Victor M, Ropper AH. *Adams and Victor's principles of neurology,* 7th ed. New York: McGraw-Hill 2001; and Shiloh R, Nutt D, Weizman A. *Essentials in clinical psychiatric pharmacotherapy.* London: Martin Dunitz, Ltd., 2001, with permission.

CLINICAL VIGNETTE

Mr. Stuart was an 85-year-old man who had a right-sided parietal stroke with resultant left-sided hemiparesis. He was admitted to a rehabilitation facility for physical and occupational therapy, but his progress was slow. In large part, this was due to the neglect of his left side and his denial of having anything wrong. He was unable to dress himself, and he had poor visuospatial skills. His refusal to participate fully in physical therapy, along with his consistent denial of any problems, eventually led to nursing home placement.

Subcortical VaD variably affects numerous regions of the brain that lie below the cortex, including the basal ganglia, thalamus, and internal capsule. The basal ganglia serve a central role in the coordination of motor movements, and they include the putamen, globus pallidus, caudate nucleus, and several brainstem nuclei. The thalamus is composed, in part, of several nuclei that integrate both motor and sensory information from the peripheral nervous system, basal ganglia, and cortical regions. The mediodorsal nuclei of the thalamus, along with hippocampal formations, are the key memory-processing centers of the brain. A complex neural feedback loop exists among the frontal cortex, basal ganglia, and thalamus to aid in the integration and regulation of motor movements, cognitive speed, mood, impulse control, and motivation. Because of these connections, subcortical damage directly affects frontal lobe function, as the typical clinical symptoms of subcortical VaD reflect; these include executive dysfunction; memory dysfunction, especially memory retrieval deficits; attentional deficits; slowed thought processing (bradyphrenia); parkinsonism (rigidity, bradykinesia, slowed gait); movement disorders; dysarthria; apathy; and depression.

Specific injury to the basal ganglia structures may result in various forms of movement disorders, including tremor, rigidity, bradykinesia, postural instability, and involuntary movements (e.g., dystonia, dyskinesia, chorea, athetosis). Thalamic injury may be reflected in dense sensory loss, and it is associated with hemiplegia when concomitant injury to the adjacent cortical motor tracts in the internal capsule occurs. Damage to some thalamic nuclei can also result in memory impairment, including Korsakoff syndrome (or thalamic amnesia), which is characterized by severe anterograde amnesia, a lack of insight, and confabulation. Binswanger disease, CADASIL, and CAA all produce clinical symptoms of subcortical VaD.

CLINICAL VIGNETTE

Mr. Lynn was a 72-year-old taxi driver with a history of hypertension. He reported several episodes of slurred speech and difficulty controlling his hand, each of which lasted only minutes. However, during one episode, he was pulled over by the police due to his erratic driving and was sent to the hospital because he could not articulate his words clearly to the officer. The medical and neurologic workup revealed lacunar infarcts. He was forced to give up his job driving a taxi, but he got a part-time job as a dispatcher. However, over the next 12 months, Mr. Lynn demonstrated increased forgetfulness and slowed motor movements. He was increasingly unable to manage his job, so he was let go. At a follow-up appointment, his physician suspected Parkinson disease, but a trial of levodopa was ineffective. Mr. Lynn became increasingly depressed, and he began spending most of his days sitting at home in front of the television. Antidepressant medication helped to improve his mood, but his wife noted that he lacked motivation to pursue his favorite hobbies, such as bowling and going to baseball games at the nearby stadium.

The presence of parkinsonism or other movement disorders is usually the most helpful symptom for distinguishing between subcortical damage and actual frontal lobe or other cortical dementias. As Chapter 1 points out, however, the distinction between cortical and subcortical dementia has been criticized as artificial because of the intimate cortical-subcortical neural connections. The differences between cortical and subcortical dementias are summarized in Table 1.2 in Chapter 1.

KEY POINT

Keep in mind that no part of the brain exists unto itself. A myriad of neural connections between brain regions, both cortical and subcortical, mean that damage to any one part will have ramifications for many others. Despite specific findings on neuropsychologic testing or the identification of specific lesions on brain scans, a prediction of the subsequent clinical picture can still be difficult.

ASSESSMENT AND DIFFERENTIAL DIAGNOSIS

Assessment of VaD follows the procedures outlined in Chapters 1 through 5, although greater diagnostic emphasis is placed on neuroimaging. The distinction between VaD and AD can be difficult, however, because the two entities can appear clinically indistinguishable and they often occur together in what is termed *mixed dementia*. Despite the fact that clinicians try to associate symptoms of dementia with strokes in VaD, a process of accumulated cerebrovascular damage, rather than single events, may account for many of the cases. Thus, VaD frequently appears to be slowly progressive like AD. Researchers have increasingly focused on the relationship between the two clinical entities; for example, vascular damage to the brain is associated with a higher risk of AD and a worse course, and both VaD and AD likely produce a central cholinergic deficit. On a gross pathologic level, the brain scans of patients with AD frequently reveal small strokes; on a microscopic level, senile plaques and neurofibrillary tangles can be found in both disorders, although they do occur with significantly greater density in AD.

Despite these similarities, several of the following factors point more toward a diagnosis of VaD: focal neurologic features, multiple vascular risk factors, brain lesions seen on neuroimaging, a more variable and less progressive course (i.e., fluctuating, stepwise deterioration), greater executive dysfunction, and less prominent memory dysfunction. These differences comprise the Hachinski Ischemic Scale, shown in Table 8.4, which assigns a score to each variable; higher scores are more consistent with VaD. Much of the information on the Hachinski Ischemic Scale can be obtained by a clinical interview and a neurologic examination. A neuropsychologic profile may help

TABLE 8.4. Hachinski Ischemic Scale

Feature[a]	Number of points
Abrupt onset	2
Stepwise deterioration	1
Fluctuating course	2
Nocturnal confusion	1
Relative preservation of personality	1
Depression	1
Somatic complaints	1
Emotional incontinence	1
History or presence of hypertension	1
History of strokes	2
Evidence of associated atherosclerosis	1
Focal neurologic symptoms	2
Focal neurologic signs	2

[a]Patient receives the number of points indicated for the presence of each feature.

Scoring: 0 to 4 points, more consistent with Alzheimer disease; 5 to 6 points, diagnosis unclear; 7 or more points, more consistent with vascular dementia.

Modified from Hachinski VC, Iliff LD, Zilhka E, et al. Cerebral blood flow in dementia. *Arch Neurol* 1975;32:632–637, with permission.

to identify VaD by revealing patchy deficits, compared with the tendency toward global impairment seen with AD. This is certainly the case in the setting of large, discrete cortical infarcts. However, one comprehensive review of neuropsychologic testing found only two areas differentiating VaD from AD—patients with VaD had greater impairment in frontal executive dysfunction and less impairment in verbal long-term memory.

NEUROIMAGING

Neuroimaging studies, such as computed tomography or magnetic resonance imaging, are helpful for identifying large strokes that lead to VaD, but the presence of cerebral atrophy, ventricular enlargement, and smaller or more diffuse cortical damage can be more difficult to interpret. One of the most controversial findings on magnetic resonance imaging is the presence of *white matter hyperintensities*, also labeled *unidentified bright objects* and *leukoariosis*. White matter hyperintensities are common subcortical findings that appear in the brains of 30% to 80% of older individuals, including those with VaD and AD. Their exact nature is controversial, but they are believed to represent small areas of ischemic damage.

Even when they are present, however, they are not always associated with cognitive impairment.

TREATMENT

As with any form of dementia, early diagnosis and treatment are important, but, in VaD, these may play a greater role because of the possibility of reducing or even arresting further vascular damage to the brain. The risk of stroke hangs over patients with VaD, increasing the morbidity and mortality over time compared with AD. The treatment of VaD involves several steps as follows:

- Primary prevention of stroke in high-risk patients;
- Secondary prevention of recurrent stroke in patients already affected;
- Consideration of the use of neuroprotective agents;
- Use of acetylcholinesterase (AChE) inhibitors.

Primary prevention seeks to reduce the chances of stroke in high-risk individuals. Lifestyle factors that may reduce risk include exercising regularly, maintaining a balanced diet, reducing obesity, and avoiding tobacco products. Control of blood pressure and glucose levels is key. Many individuals also take an aspirin daily to reduce the risk of myocardial infarction and stroke, as well as a statin medication to reduce cholesterol levels and perhaps to accrue other cardiovascular benefits. In fact, many of these interventions can reduce stroke risk by as much as 30%. In light of recent findings implicating excessive homocysteine levels in cardiovascular disease (and AD—see Chapter 6), many physicians have also begun recommending folic acid supplementation as a preventive strategy.

Secondary prevention seeks to modify the risk of recurrent stroke after previous events, and it incorporates all the strategies listed for primary prevention. Anticoagulation therapy is necessary to reduce the risk of stroke in the setting of chronic arrhythmias, such as atrial fibrillation, with warfarin (Coumadin) use conferring a 70% reduction in risk. Carotid endarterectomy may reduce the risk of stroke due to severe carotid stenosis. Another staple of stroke prevention is the use of antiplatelet agents, including aspirin, ticlopidine (Ticlid), clopidogrel (Plavix), cilostazol (Pletal), and dipyridamole (Persantine). Pentoxifylline (Trental) decreases blood viscosity and improves erythrocyte flexibility.

TIP

A review of vascular risk factors should be part of every dementia workup. When VaD is suspected or the individual has a history of stroke or multiple risk factors, involving the patient's internist and/or neurologist is critical for instituting appropriate therapy and recommending lifestyle changes. Watching and waiting in the setting of risk factors such as hypertension, carotid stenosis, and transient ischemic attacks is never an option.

Neuroprotective Agents

Over the years, several medications considered to have either protective or enhancing effects on cerebral function have been used to treat VaD. However, nearly all of the agents lack well-established efficacy in VaD, and none of these are currently recommended. Several of these medications are calcium channel blockers, such as nimodipine (Nimotop) and nicardipine (Cardene); ergoloid mesylates (Hydergine) and the ergot derivative nicergoline (Sermion); cytidinediphosphocholine (Citicoline); and the nootropic ("acting on the mind") group of amino acid compounds, including piracetam and oxiracetam.

Memantine is an N-methyl-D-aspartate receptor antagonist that has been shown to treat severe stages of AD successfully, significantly improving scores on the cognitive subscale of the Alzheimer's Disease Assessment Scale and the Mini-Mental State Examination in VaD. It is described in more detail in Chapter 7.

Acetylcholinesterase Inhibitors

Recent studies have demonstrated improvement in cognition, function, and even behavior in VaD with the use of the AChE inhibitors, including donepezil (Aricept), rivastigmine (Exelon), and galantamine (Reminyl). Given these findings, both AD and VaD likely involve central cholinergic deficits that can be ameliorated with AChE inhibitor therapy. The mechanism of these agents and the dosing strategies are covered in detail in Chapter 7.

Dementia with Lewy Bodies

Essential Concepts

- Dementia with Lewy bodies (DLB) is increasingly being recognized as a common form of dementia that is perhaps second in prevalence to Alzheimer disease (AD).
- DLB is a progressive dementia characterized by fluctuating cognitive symptoms, visual hallucinations, and parkinsonism.
- The pathologic hallmark of DLB is the presence of abnormal intracytoplasmic protein deposits called Lewy bodies (LBs).
- DLB, AD, and Parkinson disease (PD) with dementia share many clinical features, and they can be difficult to distinguish.
- Related dementias with extrapyramidal features include progressive supranuclear palsy (PSP), corticobasal degeneration (CBD), and multiple system atrophy (MSA).

Although vascular dementia has traditionally been considered the second most common form of dementia, growing evidence suggests that DLB may actually be more common. LBs are abnormal, spherical intracytoplasmic protein deposits found in both the subcortical and cortical neurons in the brains of 15% to 25% of all individuals with dementia. First identified in 1912 by the German neurologist Frederic H. Lewy, these neuronal inclusion bodies were not formally associated with a form of dementia until several seminal case reports appeared in the early 1980s. The clinical picture associated with these pathologic findings closely resembles that of both AD and vascular dementia, but, over time, researchers have begun to identify distinct features and to organize them into a more coherent diagnostic picture. Significant clinical and pathologic overlap with dementia associated with PD is also observed, leading many researchers to question whether DLB is actually a variant of PD. This chapter describes the current diagnostic picture of DLB and compares it with other major forms of dementia. Several extrapyramidal disorders that also involve dementia, including PSP, corticobasal degeneration, and MSA, are also discussed.

DIAGNOSTIC FEATURES

The initial case reports of DLB described patients with a progressive dementia that was associated with muscle rigidity and fluctuating episodes of decline in function and cognition, which were often associated with psychotic symptoms. The accumulating literature then reported what has become one of the most challenging aspects of DLB—treatment with antipsychotic or neuroleptic medications to control behavioral disturbances and psychotic symptoms can trigger episodes of acute impairment that are similar to those seen with delirium. Further clinical observation and research led to the development of consensus guidelines for DLB; these are outlined in Table 9.1. The core features of DLB, as shown in the table, are fluctuating symptoms, visual hallucinations, and parkinsonism.

Fluctuating cognitive symptoms are seen in 80% of patients with DLB, and they may involve episodes of reduced attention or alertness, somnolence, and decline in function that last from hours to weeks. During these episodes, ruling out delirium or other acute causes of mental status changes is critical. Visual hallucinations are seen in approximately 50% of patients with DLB, and these often worsen during periods of decline. The hallucinations are typically recurrent and well formed, and they may consist of animals or people. They may be associated with visuospatial impairment, visual agnosias, and occipital metabolic disturbances that are evident on positron emission tomography scans. Auditory, olfactory, and tactile hallucinations are less common, but they do have diagnostic importance as well.

CLINICAL VIGNETTE

Mr. Jacobs, a 78-year-old man, was brought to his primary care physician due to the sudden onset of confusion and daytime somnolence. He was sleeping poorly and was complaining of seeing small figures running around the house at night. When his wife was asked about recent events, she reported that they had just returned from a cruise in which Mr. Jacobs

TABLE 9.1. Consensus Criteria for the Clinical Diagnosis of Probable and Possible Dementia with Lewy Bodies

1. Progressive cognitive decline sufficient to interfere with normal social and occupational function. Prominent or persistent memory impairment may not necessarily occur in early stages, but it is evident with disease progression. Prominent neuropsychologic deficits may occur in attention, frontal/subcortical skills, and visuospatial ability.
2. Probable DLB requires at least two of the following core features, and possible DLB requires at least one: (a) fluctuating cognition with pronounced variations in attention and alertness, (b) recurrent visual hallucinations that are typically well formed and detailed, and (c) spontaneous motor features of parkinsonism.
3. Features supportive of the diagnosis include repeated falls, syncope, transient loss of consciousness, neuroleptic sensitivity, systematized delusions, hallucinations in other modalities, and depression.
4. A diagnosis of DLB is less likely in the presence of cerebrovascular disease with stroke and when another disorder that can account for the symptoms is present.

Abbreviation: DLB, dementia with Lewy bodies.
Modified from McKeith IG, Galasko D, Kosaka K, et al. Consensus guidelines for the clinical and pathologic diagnosis of dementia with Lewy bodies (DLB): report of the Consortium on DLB International Workshop. *Neurology* 1996;47:1113–1124; and McKeith IG, Perry EK, Perry RH. Report of the Second Dementia with Lewy Body International Workshop: diagnosis and treatment. Consortium on Dementia with Lewy bodies. *Neurology* 1999;53:902–905, with permission.

had an apparent stomach flu; he had been given an antiemetic agent by the ship's clinic that he took for 5 days. After thorough physical and mental status examinations, the primary care physician suspected a delirium and hospitalized Mr. Jacobs for a medical workup. Because of his increased agitation and hallucinations in the hospital, Mr. Jacobs was given several doses of haloperidol intramuscularly. Within 24 hours, he deteriorated precipitously, becoming nearly catatonic. He was taken off all of the medications and rehydrated, and, over the following 2 weeks, his mental status slowly began to clear. His function improved almost to his previous baseline over the next few weeks. However, 3 months later, his wife brought him back to the physician with recurrent hallucinations.

Although Mr. Jacobs appeared to have a delirium, he was actually in the early stages of DLB, demonstrating the typical pattern of fluctuating decline in cognition and function that was accompanied by visual hallucinations. The episode was triggered by an antiemetic medication, such as prochlorperazine (Compazine), which is actually a neuroleptic agent, and it was later exacerbated by the administration of haloperidol. As was noted, neuroleptic sensitivity is a cardinal feature of DLB.

The third core feature of DLB is parkinsonism, characterized by muscle rigidity, a stiff and slowed gait, stooped posture, bradykinesia, masked facies, and resting tremor. Parkinsonism in DLB varies in severity, and it usually manifests within a year of the cognitive deficits. However, a history of parkinsonism that predates cognitive impairment by a year or more may be more suggestive of PD associated with dementia.

Other diagnostic features include repeated falls, episodes of syncope, transient loss of consciousness, psychosis, and depression. The symptom of repeated falls may be related to the presence of subcortical brain damage that has led to extrapyramidal rigidity and bradykinesia. Extension of LB disease into the brainstem may account for the episodes of syncope. These features of DLB are seen in other forms of dementia, however, and they are often of limited diagnostic utility.

PATHOLOGIC FEATURES OF DEMENTIA WITH LEWY BODIES

The pathologic findings of DLB include cerebral atrophy and the presence of LBs in both the subcortical and cortical regions. As in AD, senile plaques are also seen, but the presence of neurofibrillary tangles is minimal. LBs are composed of a core of filamentous protein granules, including ubiquitin and α-synuclein, with a surrounding halo of neurofilaments. They are found either around the nucleus of neurons or in the dendrites. Microscopic visualization of LBs is accomplished through immunocytologic staining with antibodies to both ubiquitin and α-synuclein. Histopathologic studies have indicated that, in both DLB and PD, heavy concentrations of LBs are present in the subcortical regions, including the hypothalamus and key brainstem nuclei, such as the substantia nigra, the locus ceruleus, and the nucleus basalis of

Meynert. In patients with DLB alone, however, LBs are also seen in the cortical regions, especially the frontal and temporal lobes and the associated limbic structures.

CLASSIFICATION OF DEMENTIA WITH LEWY BODIES

As more has been learned about correlations between clinical symptoms and histopathologic findings, some researchers have classified DLB into the following types based on the location of the LBs and the degree of dementia:

1. *Diffuse LB dementia*: the LBs are located in the brainstem and cortex, and they are associated with moderate to severe dementia. Parkinsonian features are less prominent.

2. *Transitional LB dementia*: the LBs are mainly in the brainstem; fewer are in the cortex. They are associated with mild to moderate cognitive dysfunction.

3. *Brainstem LBs*: the LBs are located in the brainstem only; they are associated with PD with minimal to mild cognitive impairment.

4. *Cerebral LBs*: the LBs are found in the cerebral cortex only; they are associated with mild dementia resembling AD.

5. *Mixed LB and AD* or *LB variant of AD*: LBs, senile plaques, and neurofibrillary tangles are located in the cerebral cortex, and they are associated with a dementia similar to AD but with more pronounced impairments in attention, speech, mood, and visuospatial abilities.

✦ KEY POINT

Not only is DLB difficult to identify and distinguish from other forms of dementia, but the variety of forms of DLB can also be even more confusing. Keep in mind that the diagnostic criteria for this dementia did not appear until 1996 and that they will likely evolve over time as more is understood about the disease. Until recently, the diagnosis was limited because LBs were difficult to visualize. This process has been facilitated by the development of antiubiquitin immunostains in the past 15 years.

ASSESSMENT AND DIFFERENTIAL DIAGNOSIS

Assessment

The assessment of DLB follows the general model outlined for dementia in Chapters 1 through 5. No unique diagnostic tests for DLB exist, and, in general, neither neuroimaging nor electroencephalography is helpful. The first step should be a comparison of the clinical history with the consensus guidelines for diagnosis as given in Table 9.1. Neuropsychologic testing can provide more detailed profiles of the cognitive impairment; individuals with DLB demonstrate early impairment in memory retrieval and verbal fluency, attentional performance (e.g., digit span), visuospatial ability, and executive function. Language dysfunction is less prominent in earlier stages.

Differential Diagnosis: Parkinson Disease

Based on the subtypes of DLB, the key to diagnosis clearly lies not only in identifying characteristic symptoms but also in differentiating the condition from AD and PD with dementia. AD has been covered extensively in Chapters 6 and 7. PD is a movement disorder caused by the degeneration of a specific dopaminergic subcortical structure called the *substantia nigra*. The classic symptoms of PD are rigidity, bradykinesia, impaired gait and posture, and resting tremor. Dementia has long been a hallmark of PD, presenting clinically with the subcortical pattern described in Chapter 8. It eventually afflicts 20% to 45% of patients with PD, with the prevalence increasing with older age. Other risk factors for dementia in PD include a greater severity of motor impairment, a history of depression, and a poor response to levodopa. The rates of depression and psychosis associated with PD are as high as 40%. Both hallucinations and delusions commonly result from excessive dopaminergic activity in the mesolimbic pathways, largely as a result of antiparkinsonian medication, such as levodopa.

Twenty-five percent of individuals with PD and dementia are believed to have DLB. The consensus guidelines state that, when parkinsonism precedes symptoms of dementia by 12 months or more, the diagnosis is PD with dementia. When dementia precedes or parallels parkinsonism, the diagnosis is DLB. Clinically, distinguishing the symptoms of PD with dementia from DLB can be difficult, with several exceptions.

Compared with DLB, extrapyramidal symptoms (EPS) in PD tend to be more pronounced, and they respond to levodopa. Individuals with PD do not tend to have the fluctuating symptomatic episodes that are characteristic of DLB, and they do not demonstrate the same type of neuroleptic sensitivity, aside from the potential for increased EPS on more potent agents. In addition, myoclonus is more common in DLB, whereas tremors are more common in PD.

TREATMENT

No cure for DLB exists; the treatment involves attempts to ameliorate the clinical symptoms, including the psychosis and behavioral disturbances. As in AD and vascular dementia, DLB likely involves a central cholinergic deficiency, a possibility that explains why some individuals with DLB respond robustly to acetylcholinesterase (AChE) inhibitors. The benefits have been seen in all domains, including cognition, behavior, psychosis, and sleep disturbances.

Except for the use of AChE inhibitors, the clinician faces an immediate challenge in the treatment of agitation and psychosis because nearly 50% of patients with DLB demonstrate sensitivity to neuroleptic medications. This sensitivity is characterized by an acute decline in cognition and function, increased parkinsonism, reduced alertness and drowsiness, and a significant increase in mortality over time. These reactions usually occur within several weeks of the initiation of treatment, and they range from mild to severe, with the latter occurring in approximately one-third of sensitive individuals. Conventional antipsychotics cause the highest rate of reactions, and they should be avoided. Atypical antipsychotics are preferred because they have a lower risk, although their use must still be monitored closely for acute reactions. No one atypical agent has demonstrated clear efficacy in treating the agitation and psychosis associated with DLB, nor has the use of one been shown to offer any advantages over the use of another. Patients with PD with dementia do not demonstrate the same sensitivity to antipsychotic agents as do those with DLB, but they can experience worsening EPS. However, numerous case series indicate that individuals with PD who are treated with atypical antipsychotics can demonstrate improvements in their symptoms of both agitation and psychosis, without significant worsening of EPS. Numerous behavioral and pharmacologic strategies are still available for treating behavioral disturbances and depression in both DLB and PD; these are outlined in detail in Chapters 12 through 14.

 KEY POINT

Although some have argued that an antipsychotic agent with a low risk of EPS may be safer in DLB, clinical trials with clozapine (Clozaril), risperidone (Risperdal), olanzapine (Zyprexa), and quetiapine (Seroquel) have all demonstrated low rates of EPS when they are given in therapeutic doses to treat the agitation and psychosis associated with dementia and PD. Some clinicians argue that clozapine is the best agent for DLB because it has a more selective dopaminergic blockade that does not affect the receptors in the basal ganglia. However, this must be weighed against the potent sedative and anticholinergic effects of clozapine.

RELATED DEMENTIAS WITH EXTRAPYRAMIDAL FEATURES

The other dementias that have a clinical resemblance to DLB due to their prominent extrapyramidal features include CBD, PSP, and MSA. Although PSP and MSA both involve significant frontal lobe dysfunction, they are presented here because of their significant clinical overlap with PD. CBD shares more features with frontotemporal dementia and its variants, and thus it is presented in Chapter 10.

Progressive Supranuclear Palsy

PSP, a parkinsonian syndrome associated with dementia, is often confused with PD and other extrapyramidal syndromes. It occurs in approximately 1.39 of 100,000 people in the United States, and it may account for approximately 5% of the parkinsonian patients seen in movement disorders centers. The typical age at onset is between 50 and 70 years old, with a 7-year to 10-year survival. According to the diagnostic criteria developed by the National Institute of Neurological Disorders and Stroke and the Society for PSP, PSP is a gradually progressive disorder that begins after the age of 40. It is characterized by prominent symptoms of postural instability and falls in the first year that occur in association with vertical supranuclear gaze palsy and the slowing of vertical eye tracking movements. Histopathologic evidence of PSP includes neuronal loss, gliosis, and the presence of neurofibrillary tangles and filamentous neuropil threads in the basal ganglia and brainstem.

The early clinical symptoms of postural instability, falls, and visual disturbances are commonly followed by the development of rigidity, bradykinesia, dysphagia, and dysarthria. Visual disturbances affect 50% of patients with PSP by the end of the first year; the symptoms include diplopia, blurred vision, slowed eye movements, and vertical gaze impairment that progresses to involve all directions. Dementia associated with PSP appears in the first year in 50% of the affected individuals, and it involves memory impairment and slowed thinking. The dementia eventually affects almost all patients, but it tends to be milder than that seen in DLB and AD. The behavioral symptoms are frontal in origin, including apathy, social withdrawal, depression, and pseudobulbar palsy. Currently, no treatment for PSP exists, although 40% to 50% of patients may demonstrate mild, transient improvements in EPS on levodopa.

Multiple System Atrophy

MSA is a degenerative parkinsonian disorder that is characterized by parkinsonism, upper motor neuron impairment, cerebellar dysfunction, and dysautonomia (e.g., urinary incontinence, sexual dysfunction, orthostatic hypotension). The average age at onset is in the mid-50s, with a mean survival of 6 to 7 years. Neuronal loss and gliosis are seen throughout the basal ganglia and brainstem nuclei, with variable involvement of thalamic nuclei, olivopontocerebellar tracts, intermediolateral columns, and pyramidal tracts. The histopathologic findings include glial and, to a lesser extent, neuronal cytoplasmic inclusions that, like LBs, stain positive for the proteins ubiquitin and α-synuclein. Mild to moderate dementia with frontal lobe impairment is seen in some individuals with MSA; this typically is less severe than in DLB or AD. No effective treatment exists for MSA itself, so the current treatment strategies focus on addressing the symptom clusters, particularly the autonomic dysfunction. In general, EPS respond poorly to levodopa.

10 Frontotemporal Dementia

Essential Concepts

- Frontotemporal dementia (FTD) and its main variant, Pick disease (PiD), account for a small, but diagnostically important, group of patients with dementia.
- FTD is characterized by the early development of prominent behavioral symptoms and language disturbances, often before the advent of cognitive disturbances.
- Behavioral disturbances associated with FTD vary widely; they can include compulsive behaviors, bizarre delusions, hypersexual behaviors, apathy, unusual oral habits, and inappropriate social conduct.
- Frontal lobe symptoms are associated with many other dementia syndromes, including primary progressive aphasia and corticobasal degeneration.

The frontal lobes are unique in that they account for nearly one-third of the cerebral cortex and have great anatomic and functional diversity. For this reason, damage to frontal regions produces a spectrum of syndromes with disproportionate effects on executive function, behavioral control, and language. FTD represents a group of related dementias that have several of the following common elements: focal neuronal loss in the frontal and/or temporal lobes; cognitive impairment; and early disturbances that predominantly affect behavior, personality, and language. Given these characteristics, FTD in its early stages may closely resemble psychiatric disorders with psychotic, obsessive-compulsive, depressive, or manic features. In the middle and later stages, it is often confused with Alzheimer disease (AD). PiD, which was first described in 1892 by the neurologist Arnold Pick, is the most common form of FTD, and, until recently, it was used interchangeably with FTD. Today, it is classified as an FTD variant because of its specific pathologic findings and its typical onset at 40 to 60 years of age (range of 20 to 80 years).

CLINICAL VIGNETTE

Mrs. James was a 58-year-old woman with severe dementia who resided in a nursing home. Her clinical history indicated that she had an uneventful childhood, but she was described by her parents as an anxious child. After graduating from college with a degree in biology, she attended nursing school, eventually becoming a registered nurse in a community hospital. She married at the age of 28 and had two children over the course of the next 5 years. She and her husband began having marital problems shortly after the birth of the second child and divorced after 6 years of marriage. Mrs. James continued to work, and she got involved with the local Red Cross. Throughout her 30s and 40s, she was in good health, and she enjoyed her roles as a nurse and mother. At the age of 48, Mrs. James began having problems keeping to her schedule at work. Her children reported that she sometimes forgot to pick them up at school and that she would become uncontrollably upset when they eventually arrived home and expressed anger toward her. Fellow volunteers at the Red Cross noticed that she was quieter and that she seemed to have a hard time expressing herself. At times, she stuttered, and, when she was angry, she had a difficult time articulating her concerns. She also worried incessantly that the blood that she handled at the blood bank was contaminated, and, on several occasions, she expressed paranoid concerns to her supervisor.

At the age of 50, she had a comprehensive dementia workup, the results of which suggested the devastating diagnosis of either AD or PiD. She had already been on leave from work, but, with her mother's assistance, she went on permanent disability. As her behavior became more erratic and her cognition declined, her mother had her move into her home, and her children went to live with their father. Over the next few years, her language function deteriorated to the point where she was unable to produce basic sentences; she would instead use single words or jumbles of words to express herself. She sometimes began screaming incoherently when she could not express particular needs. She also began to demonstrate bizarre behaviors, such as hoarding cereal boxes and eating sugary breakfast cereal for every meal. Along with her progressive cognitive decline, she developed significant gait instability. Her mother became increasingly unable to care for her, largely because of the frequent bouts of agitation that required multiple psychotropic medications. At the age of 56,

Mrs. James was admitted to the dementia floor at a nearby nursing home.

The case of Mrs. James demonstrates how FTD often begins with behavioral and language disturbances in relatively young individuals and then progresses inexorably to a more global dementia.

EPIDEMIOLOGY

FTD is believed to affect 1% to 5% of all individuals with dementias, although, among individuals with early-onset dementia (younger than 65 years of age), the percentage with FTD is higher, ranging from 12% to 22%. Epidemiologic research suggests that 30% to 40% individuals with FTD may have a family history of the disorder and that having FTD in a first-degree relative may be associated with a risk of developing it that is 3.5 times greater, as well as an onset that is earlier by nearly 10 years.

DIAGNOSTIC FEATURES

Diagnostic criteria for FTD continue to evolve, and a current version of the criteria developed by a diagnostic work group for both FTD and PiD is presented in Table 10.1. The *Diag-*

TABLE 10.1. Diagnostic Criteria for Frontotemporal Dementia and Pick Disease

1. The development of behavioral or cognitive deficits manifested by either early and progressive personality and behavioral disturbances or early and progressive impairment in expressive language
2. The deficits cause significant impairment in social or occupational functioning and represent a significant decline from a previous level of functioning
3. The course is characterized by a gradual onset and continuing decline in function
4. The deficits are not due to delirium or other medical or psychiatric disease

Modified from McKhann GM, Albert MS, Grossman M, et al. Clinical and pathological diagnosis of frontotemporal dementia: report of the Work Group on Frontotemporal Dementia and Pick's Disease. *Arch Neurol* 2001;58:1803–1809, with permission.

nostic and Statistical Manual of Mental Disorders, Fourth Edition, Text Revision, criteria for PiD do not differ substantially from that of the work group. The overall clinical picture varies depending on the exact location of neuronal disease, and reviews of dementia syndromes incorporated under the heading of FTD reveal considerable diversity. Despite this heterogeneity, the two cardinal symptoms of all FTDs are language and behavioral disturbances; these present early, sometimes before overt cognitive impairment.

Language Disturbances

Language disturbances in FTD are characterized by slowed, simpler speech with word-finding difficulty, and they eventually progress to muteness. These disturbances are typically worse when the disease is disproportionately left-sided. They are associated with impairment in semantic memory or of the knowledge of particular words and objects and their meanings.

Behavioral and Personality Disturbances

Changes in behavior and personality can take various forms, but they commonly represent what would be expected from frontal and anterior temporal lobe impairment—apathy, disinhibition, and executive dysfunction. The spectrum of changes includes the following.

Apathy

The most common personality change involves an apathetic syndrome that is characterized by a lack of spontaneity, flattened affect, social withdrawal, poor insight, and a lack of concern for social etiquette, hygiene, responsibilities, and relationships.

Compulsions

Compulsive behaviors are seen in 80% of individuals with FTD. They may include hoarding objects; repetitive hand-washing; compulsive counting and checking; ritualistic arranging of objects; inflexible bathroom or hygiene habits; and repetitive questions, statements, or, later in the disease, vocalizations.

Disinhibition

Disinhibited behaviors include inappropriate social behaviors and poor judgment, such as undressing or using profanity in public, unusual dressing, unhygienic grooming or bathroom habits, and verbal or physical agitation.

Klüver–Bucy syndrome

This syndrome can result from damage to bilateral anterior temporal lobes, including the amygdala, and it is characterized by (a) hyperoral behaviors, such as craving and often overeating particular foods or insisting on the same food for most meals, especially carbohydrates, sweets, condiments, or fast food; (b) hypersexual behaviors, including inappropriate, compulsive, or intrusive sexual propositions; fondling or groping others; masturbation; and sexual acts; and (c) inappropriate, intrusive, or repetitive exploratory behavior, such as touching or grabbing objects, including unsanitary items such as garbage or feces.

Mood Disturbances

Euphoria is seen in 30% of patients with FTD, and it may mimic a manic state. Depression in FTD is atypical, being characterized by increased appetite, weight gain, irritability, and anhedonia.

Psychosis

Delusions and hallucinations commonly occur early in the course of FTD. Somatic, religious, jealous, grandiose, or bizarre delusions may occur as often as persecutory ones.

CLINICAL VIGNETTE

Mr. Cooper was a 72-year-old retired lawyer who had been recently widowed. His housekeeper noticed that his apartment had become more unkempt and that it was beginning to fill up with old newspapers and magazines. She discovered several boxes of empty soup cans stacked in one of the closets. She also noticed that Mr. Cooper had stopped his usual friendly banter with her when she cleaned and that he rarely commented on her job. She called his son frantically after she showed up on her usual cleaning day and discovered Mr. Cooper sitting in a chair and masturbating, oblivious to her presence.

PATHOLOGIC CHANGES

FTD may predominantly involve the frontal lobe, temporal lobe, or both, and it may include subcortical and parietal involvement as well. The most common manifestation of FTD generally is bilateral frontotemporal involvement, although the left hemisphere usually sustains greater atrophy. Pathologic changes in FTD include atrophy, gliosis, and spongiosis extending from the frontal into anterior temporal regions. Brain neuroimaging reveals frontal and/or temporal lobe atrophy on computed tomography or magnetic resonance imaging scans and selective hypoperfusion or hypometabolism on positron emission tomography or single photon emission computed tomography scans. Characteristic pathologic findings in PiD include spherical intracytoplasmic inclusion bodies composed of hyperphosphorylated tau protein filaments that are concentrated in the frontotemporal cortical and hippocampal regions. The atrophied areas of the brain also reveal swollen or ballooned neurons known as Pick cells. Tau protein mutations that have been mapped to chromosome 17 have been identified in familial cases of PiD. The pathologic changes in non-Pick FTD do not have any significant degree of plaques, tangles, or other neuronal inclusion bodies.

ASSESSMENT

The assessment of FTD follows the general outline presented in Chapters 1 through 5. Despite the fact that the initial presentation of FTD may be unique, the overall diagnosis is usually hampered by the progressive dementing symptoms of the disease, which often closely resemble AD. The clinical history and a thorough mental status examination, however, may reveal important clinical differences that help to distinguish FTD from AD; several of these are summarized in Table 10.2.

TABLE 10.2. **Frontotemporal Dementia Versus Alzheimer Disease**

Feature	FTD	AD
Onset	Usually 40–60 yr of age (PiD)	Usually >65 yr
Pathology	Pick bodies, Pick cells in PiD, minimal plaques and tangles	Diffuse plaques and tangles
Memory	Variable impairment	Early impairment
Language	Early impairment	Evolving aphasia
Visuospatial skills	Later impairment	Early impairment
Executive function	Early impairment	Later impairment
Behavior	Early behavior changes	Later behavioral changes

Abbreviations: AD, Alzheimer disease; FTD, frontotemporal dementia; PiD, Pick disease.

Neurologic Evaluation

A neurologic examination conducted early in the course of FTD may be entirely normal. As the disease progresses, extrapyramidal symptoms, including bradykinesia and rigidity, commonly emerge, depending on the degree of subcortical involvement and the clinical overlap with corticobasal degeneration (CBD) as described in "Related Conditions" under "Corticobasal Degeneration." Important neurologic symptoms that may emerge later in the disease course are (a) perseveration of both verbal and motor responses, including echolalia (repeating or parroting other individual's words) and echopraxia (mimicking movements), and (b) primitive reflexes that result from upper motor neuron damage to the frontal lobes and corticobulbar tracts, as seen in pseudobulbar palsy. These abnormal reflexes in adults are referred to as frontal release signs, and they include the snout or pouting reflex, the grasp reflex, the sucking reflex, the jaw-jerk reflex, the palmomental (palm-chin) reflex, and the Babinski sign (or extensor plantar reflex).

Neuropsychologic Testing

As FTD progresses, neuropsychologic testing can play a key role in identifying frontal lobe impairment, especially executive dysfunction as mediated by the dorsolateral regions. Two bedside neuropsychologic tests that have been developed to assess dorsolateral frontal lobe function include the Frontal Assessment Battery and the Executive Interview. The Frontal Assessment Battery is a 10-minute test composed of six subtests measuring various skills, such as conceptualization, mental flexibility, motor programming, sensitivity to interference, inhibitory control, and autonomy. The patient is asked to carry out a simple task to assess each skill. The Executive Interview measures similar skills, but it also incorporates frontal release signs and shortened versions of several neuropsychologic tasks. The "Suggested Reading" section at the end of the book has references for these tests.

Discrete neuropsychologic tests that can identify impairment in executive dysfunction include word fluency tests; the Wisconsin Card Sorting Test (WCST); the Trail-Making Test, Part B (TMT-B); and the subtests of the Luria Motor Battery. In word fluency tests, the subject is asked to generate a list of items in particular categories, such as animals or foods. The WCST requires an individual to sort cards in piles based on a specific category that is changed midway through the task. In the TMT-B, an individual is asked to draw lines between alternating, successive letters and numbers scattered on a page. Both the WCST and the TMT-B require subjects to shift their mental set between different rules or categories for a successful performance. The tasks from the Luria Motor Battery involve having the patient imitate a series of sequential hand movements. Impairment in all these tests is manifested by inflexible mental strategies, inappropriate or disinhibited responses, and perseverated actions. Numerous neuropsychologic tests can also identify impairments in other aspects of frontal lobe function, including motor behavior, visual tracking, smell identification, and inhibitory control.

Quick Clinical Assessment of Frontal Lobe Function

If one is evaluating a patient in a clinic, the following tests, several of which come from the Frontal Assessment Battery and the Executive Interview, can be used to assess frontal lobe function:

Abstracting. Ask the patient to tell how an apple and a banana are alike. In frontal lobe impairment, look for a failure to determine conceptual similarity (e.g., both are fruits); instead, he or she might deny any similarities or focus on less abstract and more concrete responses (e.g., aspects of shape and color).

Word fluency. Ask the patient to list as many animals or words beginning with the same letter as he or she can in 60 seconds. Individuals without impairment should be able to list at least 10.

Motor programming.
- *Luria Hand Sequence.* Ask the patient to observe you and to imitate the following three hand movements in their exact order: (a) make a fist and hit it on the table, (b) open the hand and hit the table again with the side of the hand, and (c) slap the table with the hand, palm side down. Look for a failure to imitate and to organize the sequence and for perseverated movements.
- Tap a pattern with your hand and ask the patient to repeat it.
- Draw a series of loops and ask the patient to copy it.

Disinhibition.
- Check for frontal release signs. Extend your hand to the patient, but ask him or her not to shake it. Look for the patient's inability to inhibit a natural response. Ask the patient to tap only one time after each time you tap twice. Look for perseverated behaviors.
- Consider asking a consulting neuropsychologist for a copy of the TMT-B to administer.

COURSE

Both FTD and the PiD variant follow a time course similar to that of AD, with progressive deterioration over 2 to 10 years until eventual death. Individuals become severely aphasic and then mute, with severe cognitive impairment and often tremor and motor rigidity.

TREATMENT

Treatment of FTD itself has not been well established, in part because of the relatively small size of identified cohorts. The basis of treatment may rest on neurotransmitter deficiencies identified through decreased cholinergic and serotonergic receptor binding in the affected cortical regions. For example, symptoms of FTD, including carbohydrate craving, overeating with weight gain, depression, impulse dyscontrol, and compulsive behaviors, may reflect underlying serotonergic dysfunction. Small studies of selective serotonin reuptake inhibitor antidepressants have shown improvement of several of these symptoms in FTD (see Chapter 14 for specific agents and dosing). Although the presence of cholinergic deficits would suggest that use of acetylcholinesterase inhibitors would also benefit patients with FTD, to date, few data support their use. Behavioral disturbances and depressive symptoms associated with FTD and its related conditions should respond to the variety of behavioral, environmental, and pharmacologic strategies outlined in Chapters 12 through 14.

RELATED CONDITIONS

Several degenerative neurologic conditions share both clinical and pathologic features with FTD in general and PiD in particular. In addition, in common with dementia with Lewy bodies, these conditions have pathologic involvement of subcortical regions with associated extrapyramidal symptoms.

Primary Progressive Aphasia

Primary progressive aphasia (PPA) is characterized by an evolving expressive aphasia with nonfluent speech and word-finding difficulty. As in PiD, the language disturbances progress to eventual muteness. Although memory disturbances are not prominent early in the course of PPA, many cases progress to a more generalized dementia within several years. Autopsy studies usually find frontotemporal lobe neuronal loss and gliosis, with microscopic findings similar to those in PiD.

Corticobasal Degeneration

CBD, also called cortical-basal ganglionic degeneration, is a neurodegenerative condition characterized by the progressive development of asymmetric parkinsonism with limb rigidity and stiff gait, apraxia, and cortical sensory loss; less common symptoms include the alien hand phenomenon (complex and seemingly purposeful hand movements without cognitive control) and reflex myoclonus. The extrapyramidal motor symptoms are typically unresponsive to levodopa. Within 2 to 3 years, most affected individuals go on to demonstrate dementia that is associated with behavioral and language disturbances. Nearly 50% of affected individuals initially present with frontal lobe dysfunction. In some cases, personality changes and language disturbances may present before the motor symptoms. Given this clinical picture, the differential diagnosis is wide, including AD, PD, and FTD or PiD. Because decreased dexterity in a hand is often a presenting symptom in CBD, *amyotrophic lateral sclerosis* (i.e., Lou Gehrig disease) is sometimes suspected, and it, in fact, has demonstrated some symptomatic overlap with both CBD and FTD.

Neuroimaging in CBD typically reveals focal frontal and sometimes parietal atrophy and hypoperfusion, often asymmetrically. Similarly, autopsy studies typically find asymmetric frontal and parietal neuronal loss and gliosis. Pathologic findings are usually consistent with PiD, including ballooned neurons and inclusion bodies positive for tau protein. Neurofibrillary tangles are also seen in the affected cortical, subcortical, and brainstem regions.

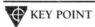 **KEY POINT**

Multiple studies have found significant overlap between FTD, PPA, and CBD. In one case series, 35 individuals with CBD all developed either FTD or PPA, most within 6 months of presenting with either an extrapyramidal movement disorder or a behavioral or language impairment. Distinguishing among these clinical entities can be difficult, and collaboration among neurologists, psychiatrists, and neuropsychologists is required.

SECONDARY FRONTOTEMPORAL DEMENTIA

Numerous medical conditions can produce dementia syndromes with predominant frontal lobe impairment. These include the following: Huntington disease, Wilson disease, multiple sclerosis, human immunodeficiency virus infection, Creutzfeldt–Jakob disease, and alcohol abuse. These conditions are discussed in more detail in Chapter 11.

Dementia Associated with Medical Conditions

> **Essential Concepts**
> - Various medical conditions can cause dementia or can worsen the existing cognitive impairment caused by other major forms of dementia.
> - The clinical symptoms of dementia due to medical conditions vary widely depending on the nature of the brain injury, but they may be reversible with early treatment.

Medical conditions that cause dementia vary widely, including direct trauma to the brain; neoplasm; toxic exposure; oxygen deprivation; vitamin deficiencies; central nervous system (CNS) infections; and chronic neurologic, metabolic, endocrine, and inflammatory diseases. The goal of this chapter is not to present every possible condition that can lead to dementia in detail; that is the subject of a whole volume. Rather, this chapter presents the major categories of medical conditions and details several of the most common found in each. The focus is on those conditions that can actually cause a dementia because innumerable medical conditions can cause transient confusion, neurologic symptoms, psychosis, and behavioral disturbances but not the enduring cognitive impairment that would constitute a dementia. A complete list of dementia types can be found in Table 1.1 in Chapter 1.

The guiding criteria for the dementia subtypes described in this chapter come from the *Diagnostic and Statistical Manual of Mental Disorders*, Fourth Edition, Text Revision, (DSM-IV-TR) diagnostic category of "dementia due to other general medical conditions." The basic criteria for this diagnosis are identical to those for the major forms of dementia (see Chapter 1). They include (a) the development of multiple cognitive deficits manifested by memory impairment and one or more of the following: aphasia, apraxia, agnosia, and executive dysfunction; and (b) these symptoms lead to significant social and occupational impairment and represent a significant decline from a previous level of functioning. The third criterion is unique, requiring that evidence from the history, physical examination, or laboratory findings must indicate that the cognitive impairment is a direct physiologic consequence of a general condition other than Alzheimer disease (AD) or cerebrovascular disease.

 TIP

In older individuals, snap diagnoses of AD or vascular dementia (VaD) are often made without a recognition of the critical underlying medical conditions that may actually be the cause of the dementia. Treatment of these conditions can lead to improvement in, or even the reversal of, symptoms. With this in mind, the importance of a complete medical workup in every case of dementia should be obvious.

CLINICAL VIGNETTE

Mrs. Taylor was a 93-year-old woman with a 6-month history of cognitive decline and behavioral disturbances. She was always considered a relatively bright woman, but now her son described her thinking as "slowed down." In the dining room of the assisted-living facility, she would sometimes yell at wait staff and use obscene language. She also fell several times. A routine medical workup was unrevealing, and Mrs. Taylor was tentatively diagnosed with AD. She was started on an acetylcholinesterase inhibitor and an antidepressant medication. Her irritability and intermittent agitation continued without improvement. She began to have periods of increased confusion, and she was eventually hospitalized with delirium. In the hospital, Mrs. Taylor was found to have hypercalcemia, and a further workup revealed the source to be a parathyroid adenoma. Despite the risks, she underwent surgery to remove the growth. Her calcium levels normalized, and, over the next 3 months, her cognition and behavior improved significantly.

In the case of Mrs. Taylor, the clues that pointed to the possibility of an underlying medical cause included the rather precipitous onset of cognitive impairment and a history of falls and periods of confusion. Unfortunately, the reversible cause of dementia was missed in the initial workup. This mistake is not uncommon, especially when clinicians are so used to seeing AD or VaD that they assume that every case of cognitive impairment must be caused by one or the other. However, several factors in the clinical presentation of any dementia may indicate a higher likelihood of an underlying medical cause. These are listed in Table 11.1.

The case reveals a pattern of frontotemporal and subcortical symptoms common to many dementias caused by medical conditions. The spectrum of these symptoms includes the following:

- Personality changes: apathy, disinhibition, impulsivity, lability;
- Early behavioral disturbances: agitation, aggression, inappropriate behaviors;
- Psychiatric symptoms: depression, mania, psychosis;
- Movement disorders: extrapyramidal or parkinsonian symptoms;
- Cognitive decline: memory impairment, bradyphrenia (slowed thinking).

The preponderance of early behavioral disturbances *without* prominent language impairment may help distinguish a

TABLE 11.1. Factors Pointing to Higher Likelihood of Dementia Due to a Medical Condition

Sudden or precipitous onset of dementia
Rapid progression of cognitive decline
Young age at onset (<65 yr)
Recent major medical illness
Chronic medical illness
Recent unexplained illness
Recent cancer chemotherapy or radiation treatment
Recent surgery
Family history of dementia subtype
Head trauma
Substance abuse (especially alcohol)
History of occupational exposure to potentially toxic substances
Prominent frontotemporal and/or subcortical symptoms
Recent onset of focal neurologic symptoms without evidence of stroke (e.g., parkinsonism, ataxia, myoclonus, incontinence, paraesthesias, weakness)
Recent episodes of confusion or delirium

dementia caused by a medical condition from that of a frontotemporal dementia.

DEMENTIA CAUSED BY STRUCTURAL OR TRAUMATIC INJURY

As Chapter 5 describes, brain imaging is a key diagnostic component to the dementia workup. Because AD typically has unremarkable findings on computed tomography or magnetic resonance imaging (MRI), the purpose of neuroimaging often is to rule out specific medical conditions in the brain, including tumors, trauma, bleeding, and strokes. This section covers dementia caused by neoplastic tumors, traumatic brain injury (TBI), chronic subdural hematomas, normal pressure hydrocephalus, and brain injury caused by anoxia and surgery. The effects of stroke are covered in Chapter 8 on VaD.

Neoplastic Tumors

Both primary and metastatic brain tumors can cause dementia. The clinical course is highly variable depending on the location and type of growth and the success of treatment. Neoplastic growths in the brain can arise from the brain parenchyma itself and from surrounding tissues, such as the cerebral vessels and meninges. Benign meningiomas are the most common brain tumor in the elderly, followed by malignant gliomas as the second most common. Pituitary adenomas and metastatic disease make up a smaller percentage of the cerebral neoplasms encountered.

Cognitive impairment caused by neoplastic growths stems from damage or pressure to regions of the brain that is caused by tumor infiltration and destruction, with subsequent hemorrhage, occlusion of vessels, compression or mass effect, increased intracranial pressure, and hydrocephalus. The specific symptoms vary by which lobe of the brain is affected, and they are reviewed in Table 8.3 in Chapter 8. As a result of a paraneoplastic syndrome, dementia may also be caused by the distant effects of a malignancy that is outside the CNS. *Limbic encephalitis* is a paraneoplastic syndrome that is most commonly associated with small cell lung carcinoma and Hodgkin disease and is manifested primarily by memory disturbances and psychiatric symptoms.

TIP

Dementia associated with neoplasms of the brain can present insidiously, with the symptoms of cognitive and behavioral decline that are seen in many other forms of dementia. This is especially true of benign meningiomas that may grow for periods of years to decades without causing the focal neurologic symptoms that would trigger investigation. As every section of this chapter emphasizes, always get a brain scan when conducting an evaluation of dementia.

Depending on the success of treatment, the dementia that is caused by brain neoplasms or paraneoplastic disease is potentially reversible. A small percentage of cancer survivors may, however, develop cerebral demyelination months to years after receiving chemotherapy (e.g., methotrexate, cyclosporine) or brain radiation. Typical symptoms in these individuals include dementia, apathy, and motor disturbances.

CLINICAL VIGNETTE

Mr. Schwartz, a 78-year-old retired banker, fell and broke a hip while working in his garage. After surgery, he was admitted to a rehabilitation facility where he was noted to be confused and irritable. At times, he would direct angry outbursts at staff, and he began alienating friends and family members with his verbally abusive language and labile moods. A psychiatric consultation suggested that Mr. Schwartz was depressed and that he possibly had early AD. He was started on an antidepressant medication, and, within 3 weeks, he demonstrated mild improvement. An antipsychotic medication was added to the therapeutic regimen because of his ongoing verbally abusive behaviors. Several days after being started on the antipsychotic, Mr. Schwartz had a tonic-clonic seizure. A brain computed tomography scan revealed a large mass consistent with a glioblastoma multiforme. Palliative radiation therapy and control of the cerebral edema resulted in significant behavioral improvements.

In the case of Mr. Schwartz, the evolving symptoms of dementia and agitation in a man who had been cognitively intact were not attributed to a brain malignancy until a seizure occurred. Despite his poor prognosis, Mr. Schwartz's cognitive and behavioral symptoms benefited significantly from the treatment.

Traumatic Brain Injury

TBI affects an estimated two to three million individuals in the United States each year, and it is the leading cause of cognitive impairment in young adults. The key elements that define TBI include physical brain injury with a loss or change of consciousness, posttraumatic amnesia, and evidence of trauma on the clinical or physical examination. Because motor vehicle accidents and falls are the two most common causes of TBI, the following two peaks in prevalence are observed: in young adults 15 to 25 years old, with a 3:1 male-to-female ratio, and then after the age of 65. Motor vehicle accidents are more common than falls in young adults, whereas the reverse is true for the elderly. Alcohol intoxication is often a factor in TBI in both young and old.

TBI can be classified by *the type of injury* (penetrating the skull and brain versus nonpenetrating, blunt trauma), the *extent of the injury* (focal versus diffuse), the *time course of the injury* (primary damage from injury or secondary damage from edema, hemorrhage, hematoma, increased intracranial pressure, infection, seizures, or changes in neurotransmitter function), and *the severity* (mild, moderate, severe). Nonpenetrating or closed injuries, which are more common, often result from rapid acceleration and deceleration in motor vehicle accidents or the blunt force of an object. Because the brain "floats" within the skull, it becomes slightly mobile during trauma; the injury may therefore occur at the site of impact (coup) and a contralateral (contrecoup) site as well, often in the anterior and inferior regions of the frontal and temporal lobes that sit on top of the bony protuberances in the skull. Diffuse brain injury results from more severe twisting, stretching, or shearing movements of the brain that damage the neuronal axons. Most TBIs are mild, meaning that the loss of consciousness is brief and that the posttraumatic amnesia lasts less than 60 minutes. Severe injury involves the loss of consciousness for hours to days and posttraumatic amnesia lasting more than 24 hours; moderate injuries lie somewhere in between. The Glasgow Coma Scale, a 15-point scale that measures ocular, verbal, and motor responsiveness, is frequently used in the acute setting to rate the severity of TBI.

In addition to the factors already listed, the outcome of any given TBI depends on the location of the injury; the age of the patient; his or her premorbid personality characteristics; his or her social, family, and financial resources; and his or her psychiatric history. Factors such as a lower initial postinjury score on the Glasgow Coma Scale, advanced age, a longer duration of the loss of consciousness and posttraumatic amnesia, a longer length of hospitalization, and a history of psychiatric problems and substance abuse portend a slower and more difficult recovery.

Mild TBI can result in a postconcussive syndrome that is characterized by short-term memory impairment; slowed cognitive processing; decreased concentration; and neurologic symptoms, including headache, blurred vision, and dizziness. Individuals may also experience depression, anxiety, and posttraumatic stress disorder. These symptoms can last for months to years after the injury, but they usually improve with time and appropriate treatment. More severe TBI can result in both focal neurologic symptoms and evidence of diffuse neuronal injury, including deficits in memory-processing speed and efficiency, executive dysfunction, language impairment, behavioral disturbances (e.g., impulsivity, agitation, irritability, apathy), and depression. Disruptions in emotional regulation may represent the primary physical effects of the brain injury, as well as the psychologic reactions to the trauma.

The initial treatment of TBI is devoted to the acute effects of the injury, with the goal of reducing permanent damage. Acute recovery is followed by aggressive physical, occupational, and speech therapy, as well as any appropriate psychiatric or psychologic treatment. Cognitive and neurologic impairment often improves with therapy, although, with severe injury, usually areas of residual impairment are present. Anticonvulsant medications are frequently used for seizure prophylaxis after TBI, and they may help in mood regulation and the control of aggression and agitation. Individuals with behavioral disturbances after TBI may benefit from treatment with antipsychotic medications, although some patients demonstrate increased sensitivity to their side effects. Antidepressants and anxiolytics are used for mood disturbances.

An important TBI syndrome associated with dementia that is seen in the elderly is *chronic subdural hematoma* (SDH). Although SDHs can occur acutely after injury, they can also present chronically, producing fluctuating symptoms of confusion, apathy, lethargy, memory impairment, and executive dysfunction. More than two-thirds of SDHs occur after the age of 60, and nearly one-third of the affected individuals present with no history of trauma. Elderly individuals with gait disturbances, frequent falls, and anticoagulant therapy are at greatest risk for SDHs. The diagnosis is made by contrast-enhanced brain computed tomography or MRI, the latter of which is superior. Some SDHs can resorb over time, but others may persist; these may even become cystic structures that are surrounded by fibrous membranes. When chronic SDHs do not resolve quickly and they cause both cognitive decline and/or focal neurologic symptoms, the treatment of choice is surgical evacuation.

The final form of TBI worth mentioning is *dementia pugilistica*, which is seen in boxers late into their careers or even years afterward. Dementia pugilistica is characterized by parkinsonism, personality changes, and dementia. The brain injury caused by repeated blows to the head during boxing matches is assumed to be the source of the dementia. Dementia pugilistica is associated with cerebellar scarring and substantia nigra degeneration. The pathologic findings include neurofibrillary tangles and β-amyloid deposits.

Normal Pressure Hydrocephalus

Normal pressure hydrocephalus (NPH) is characterized by the symptom triad of progressive dementia, gait disturbance, and urinary incontinence. The dementia symptoms include slowed thinking or bradyphrenia, memory impairment, and executive dysfunction. NPH represents less than 2% of all dementias, and the average age at onset is between 60 and 70 years. The disease process involves impaired circulation of the cerebrospinal fluid (CSF), with resultant ventricular dilation and the demyelination of the periventricular white matter. The intracranial pressure is normal, most likely representing the achievement of a state of equilibrium between the formation and absorption of CSF despite ongoing neuronal damage. However, increased CSF pressure can be encountered in similar forms of hydrocephalic dementia. The underlying cause of NPH is either idiopathic or secondary to trauma, infection, or subarachnoid hemorrhage. Idiopathic NPH may evolve slowly over months to years, whereas NPH caused by acute causes has a more rapid onset.

Treatment of NPH may involve serial spinal taps to drain the CSF, but, more typically, it necessitates the placement of a ventriculoperitoneal shunt. The rates of improvement after shunting range from 30% to 50%, while those of complications, including more severe impairment and death, average more than 40%. Predictors of a better outcome after shunting include a known cause of the NPH, a shorter history of cognitive decline, predominant gait disturbance, and higher CSF outflow resistance.

Postanoxic and Postoperative Dementia

Both acute and chronic oxygen deprivation to the brain can result in brain damage and a dementia syndrome that is characterized by confusion, impaired memory, apathy, irritability, and somnolence. Individuals who survive severe anoxia caused by sustained cardiac or respiratory arrest or other traumatic causes often have profound residual neuropsychologic impairment. Less severe cognitive impairment can sometimes result from a variety of acute and chronic conditions that produce cerebral hypoxia, including brief cardiopulmonary failure, inadequate surgical ventilation, open heart surgery, sleep apnea, bradycardia, chronic obstructive pulmonary disease, congestive heart failure, anemia, and hyperviscous or hypercoagulable states.

Findings of cognitive impairment associated with coronary artery bypass surgery (CABG), which is performed on half a million Americans every year, have been a source of particular concern in the medical literature. Mild impairment in memory processing, mathematical ability, complex planning, ability to follow directions, and mood regulation has been seen in a significant number of individuals after CABG, with individuals who are older and more medically compromised having the greatest risk. One longitudinal study demonstrated cognitive impairment on discharge in 53% of CABG patients, a figure that decreased to 36% at 6 weeks and 24% at 6 months but then rose to 42% in those individuals seen at follow-up 5 years later. Even after the natural rate of dementia was taken into consideration, the rates in the post-CABG group were two to three times greater than expected. The speculation is that this impairment could be caused by one of several of the following factors: (a) cerebral microemboli that occur during aortic manipulation and cross-clamping, (b) the use of the cardiopulmonary bypass pump, (c) cerebral hypoperfusion, and (d) the effects of the anesthesia. Surgical procedures that minimize or eliminate aortic manipulation and clamping and off-pump CABG are ways to reduce these factors during CABG. However, these do not eliminate the potential negative effects of anesthesia on cognition that have been found in elderly patients after both cardiac and noncardiac surgery. These findings remain controversial, and many researchers have argued that the negative cognitive influences of depression, anxiety, and the use of sedative-hypnotics are not fully accounted for when older postsurgical patients are studied.

⊕ KEY POINT

Although the prognosis of postanoxic or postoperative dementia can never be clearly predicted, reasons for optimism and encouraging aggressive rehabilitation always exist. For most of the affected individuals, the deficits are mild to moderate, and they will improve within the first year. Cognitive rehabilitation, when it is available, can benefit the individual's memory and other cognitive skills. When an individual has cognitive impairment that seems out of proportion to cerebral damage, comorbid depression; medication effects, especially those from narcotics and steroids; and an underlying progressive dementia, such as AD, should always be suspected. Cerebral injury can sometimes trigger or accelerate the deterioration in AD.

DEMENTIA CAUSED BY MEDICATIONS, SUBSTANCES, AND TOXINS

When an individual is being evaluated for dementia secondary to medications, substance abuse, or toxic exposure, differentiating between the acute effects of overexposure, intoxication, or withdrawal and the chronic effects of exposure is critical. For most individuals, the acute effects remit when the offending substance is withdrawn, but they can return with repeated exposure. The changes in mental status caused by acute overexposure range from mild confusion to frank delirium and psychosis and ultimately to coma and death. Dementia syndromes, conversely, represent the more insidious, often permanent effects of chronic exposure that sometimes worsen after abstinence. These factors, as well as the general criteria for dementia stated in the introduction, are captured by the DSM-IV-TR diagnostic category of *substance-induced persisting dementia*. Table 11.2 contains a list of substances that can cause dementia.

Medications on the list come from a range of pharmacologic categories, but a common link among many of them are their effects on CNS receptors, including γ-aminobutyric acid agonism and cholinergic (muscarinic) antagonism. γ-Aminobutyric acid receptors have multiple sites of action, and they serve an inhibitory role on cerebral function when they are activated by sedative-hypnotics (e.g., benzodiazepines, barbi-

TABLE 11.2. Medications, Substances, and Toxins Associated with Cognitive Impairment and Dementia

Medications
  Anticholinergics and antispasmodics
    Atropine, benztropine (Cogentin), dicyclomine (Bentyl, others), hyoscyamine (component in Donnatal, Donnagel), scopolamine (Pamine, others)
    See also Table 3.2.
  Anticonvulsants
    Divalproex sodium (Depakote, Depakene), carbamazepine (Tegretol), phenytoin (Dilantin)
  Antipsychotics
    Chlorpromazine (Thorazine)
    Thioridazine (Mellaril)
  Azathioprine (Imuran)
  Clonidine (Catapres)
  Digitalis (Digoxin)
  Disulfiram (Antabuse)
  Lithium (Eskalith, Lithobid)
  Sedative-hypnotics
    Barbiturates, benzodiazepines, chloral hydrate
  Tricyclic antidepresants
Substances
  Alcohol
  Inhalants (solvents)
Toxins
  Gases (carbon monoxide, carbon disulfide)
  Metals (e.g., aluminum, arsenic, copper, lead, manganese, mercury)
  Industrial solvents
  Organophosphate pesticides

turates), anticonvulsants, and alcohol. The therapeutic and eventually intoxicating properties of these substances clearly illustrate their depressive effects on CNS function. The long-term use of these agents can result in more insidious, but equally disabling, impairments in cognition and function, especially in individuals with preexisting dementia.

Similar degrees of cognitive impairment can result from the potent anticholinergic effects of many commonly used medications, especially when they are used in combination (see Table 3.2 for a complete list). Atropine and its analogues, which are used for their antispasmodic effects, are the prototypical anticholinergic agents. The tricyclic antidepressants and the conventional antipsychotics chlorpromazine (Thorazine) and thioridazine (Mellaril) are examples of psychotropic medications with potent anticholinergic effects. As Chapter 12 describes, these effects limit their use in older populations. In general, the dementia syndromes produced by all of these medications tend to reverse after discontinuation.

Alcohol Dementia

Alcohol abuse is a major health problem in the United States, accounting for a variety of comorbid medical and psychiatric conditions. Cognitive problems result from the direct toxic effects of alcohol on the liver, brain, and other organs and from the secondary effects of alcohol abuse (e.g., malnutrition, vitamin deficiencies, an increased risk of stroke and head injury). The concept of *alcohol dementia* is controversial because of the difficulty in separating the role of alcohol from that of other comorbid conditions and due to the lack of specific neuropathologic findings. Despite this controversy, the risk of dementia is clearly increased in alcoholics, and alcohol may play a negative role in the development of dementia in 4% to more than 20% of individuals with dementia.

The best studied dementia associated with alcohol abuse is the *Wernicke–Korsakoff syndrome*, which is characterized by the following two stages: the acute onset of confusion, gaze palsy, nystagmus, and ataxia (collectively referred to as *Wernicke encephalopathy*); without treatment, it may progress to a permanent dementia syndrome involving severe retrograde and anterograde amnesia and confabulation (termed *Korsakoff syndrome*). The Wernicke–Korsakoff syndrome is attributed to thiamine deficiency and the consequent damage to the cerebral mammillary bodies and adjacent thalamic nuclei (however, Korsakoff syndrome, as a separate entity, can have other causes). Rapid treatment with thiamine supplementation may reverse the symptoms to varying degrees, but a delay in intervention frequently leads to permanent dementia in 80% of individuals.

In contrast to Wernicke–Korsakoff syndrome, alcohol dementia involves mild to moderate memory impairment, slowed cognitive processing, and executive dysfunction that may resemble frontal lobe impairment. The individual's language function is typically intact. Neuroimaging studies and corresponding pathologic findings demonstrate neuronal atrophy with sulcal widening in the frontal and mediotemporal lobes, ventricular dilation, the loss of hippocampal pyramidal cells, and the degeneration of the cerebellar vermis. The pathologic changes have not always correlated with the degree of cognitive impairment.

Because some researchers have argued that alcohol dementia and Wernicke–Korsakoff syndrome may both result from thiamine deficiency and that they vary only in degree, the use of thiamine and multivitamin supplementation are reasonable first steps in the treatment of suspected alcohol dementia. Obviously, abstinence from alcohol is critical, and this goal may necessitate inpatient detoxification, followed by intensive substance abuse therapy. The mainstay of treatment of alcohol abuse remains supportive therapy, especially in the setting of 12-step groups, such as Alcoholics Anonymous. If true abstinence is achieved, the prognosis for both Wernicke–Korsakoff syndrome and alcohol dementia is variable, but improvement is possible.

A dementia syndrome associated with alcohol abuse in older men is *Marchiafava–Bignami disease*, which causes demyelination of the corpus callosum and the adjacent white matter. The associated neurologic symptoms include incontinence, dysarthria, frontal release signs, hemispheric disconnection, seizures, and personality changes with apathy or agitation.

Toxic Metal and Gas Exposure

Dementia caused by toxic metals or gases requires either massive acute exposure or significant long-term exposure to high levels of dust, fumes, or liquid through inhalation, skin absorption, or ingestion. Occupational exposure is one of the most common settings in which this occurs. Acute poisoning can cause neurologic symptoms, mental status changes, and organ damage that require emergent intervention, usually as a result of the primary damaging effects of the substance itself. Permanent dementia may also result from such poisoning, often secondary to an anoxic injury, stroke, or head injury associated with the exposure. In general, dementia caused by toxic metal exposure has become rare because of improved occupational safety regulations and the elimination of environmental hazards. Consequently, few dementia workups will hinge on a heavy metal screen.

However, obtaining an employment history and probing for possible occupational exposures to toxic metals or other substances are important. Occupations with the potential for hazardous exposure include mining; smelting or foundry work; welding; plumbing; construction work; extermination or fumigation; agricultural work involving proximity to pesticides, herbicides, or fungicides; and manufacturing or craftsmanship work with metals, glass, ceramics, paints, varnishes or stains, dental amalgams, automotive parts, chemicals, or batteries. Metals associated with toxic exposure in these and other settings include lead, mercury, manganese, arsenic, copper, chromium, nickel, tin, iron, zinc, antimony, bismuth, barium, silver, gold, platinum, lithium, thallium, and aluminum. Some of the more common exposures are discussed in this section.

Other toxic substances that can cause neurologic impairment and, more rarely, cognitive disturbances from overexposure include carbon monoxide, carbon disulfide, organophosphate insecticides, and numerous industrial solvents (e.g., toluene, hexacarbons, hydrocarbons). Poisoning can also result from the intentional inhalation or sniffing of vapors from volatile solvents to get "high." Commonly abused solvents include toluene, halogenated hydrocarbons, benzene, and acetone, which are found in common products such as glues, gasoline, spray paints, and cleaning fluids. Brain damage from intentional inhalation results only after significant long-term exposure.

TIP

Prolonged exposure to some metals leads to their accumulation in tissues such as the kidney, brain, bone, and liver, with relatively slow rates of metabolic clearance. Initial manifestations of toxicity often include neurologic symptoms, such as an ascending peripheral neuropathy, visual disturbances, and weakness. When toxic exposure is suspected, obtain a heavy metal screen, but check with the relevant laboratory to determine which metals are included in the screen. Separate blood, urine, and even hair samples are sometimes needed to get a complete screen. The first step in treatment is to identify and to eliminate the route of exposure. If this can be done and the symptoms are not severe, the body will eventually clear the metal. Adjunctive treatment, especially with heavy exposure or severe symptoms such as dementia, involves the administration of chelating agents to bind the metal, forming a more stable, less toxic, and more excretable compound. Common chelating agents include succimer with ^{99m}Tc-dimercaptosuccinic acid, known as DMSA; calcium ethylenediaminetetraacetic acid, known as EDTA; penicillamine; and dimercaprol.

Chronic *lead* poisoning, or plumbism, is more of a concern with children who might be exposed to environmental lead, usually in the form of paint chips or dust from old houses. In adults, sources of chronic lead exposure are less common, but they may include contamination from lead-glazed ceramics; lead paint; and occupational work with lead, including metal and ceramic work, construction, and plumbing. Symptoms of lead poisoning in children include cognitive impairment, developmental delay, neurologic symptoms, and behavioral disturbances. These symptoms are less predictable in adults. The risk of an actual dementia syndrome is present only when blood levels exceed 80 μg per dL.

Mercury is a particularly poisonous metal with numerous industrial uses. It is present in the following three forms: elemental mercury, inorganic mercury salts (e.g., mercuric chloride), and organic mercury compounds (e.g., methylmercury). Exposure can occur through oral ingestion, the inhalation of vapors, or transdermally. Historically, mercury poisoning was seen in hatmakers, who used mercury to process felt for men's hats in the 19th and early 20th century (as illustrated by the character of the Mad Hatter in Lewis Carroll's *Alice in Wonderland*). Chronic exposure to mercury is associated with neurologic impairment (headache, fatigue, ataxia, paresthesias, visual and hearing impairment, tremor), skin eruptions, renal toxicity, cognitive impairment, depression, and psychosis.

 KEY POINT

The presence of a mercury-based amalgam in dental fillings has not been associated with dementia or any other medical problems; the concern regarding exposure is for individuals creating or preparing such amalgams.

Manganese, a trace element, is an essential mineral in skin, nerve, bone, and cartilage formation. Manganese toxicity is rare, but it may occur from overexposure to industrial or pharmaceutical sources, including manganese ore and dust from mining and the manufacture of metal alloys, batteries, varnish, fungicides, and gasoline additives. Chronic manganese overexposure over several years has been seen mainly in miners, and it is associated with "manganese madness," which is characterized by cognitive impairment, psychosis, and behavioral disturbances consistent with frontal lobe impairment (e.g., mood lability, compulsive behaviors), followed by extrapyramidal symptoms.

Toxic exposure to *arsenic* and arsenic compounds can result from inhalation in industrial work, including the smelting industry, and the production of microelectronics, pesticides, fungicides, wood preservatives, coloring agents, and paints. Recently, much concern has been expressed concerning the health risks posed to children due to the use of pressure-treated lumber containing chromated copper arsenate, an arsenic-containing preservative, in playground equipment, decks, and picnic tables. Arsenic may also be used in intentional poisonings. Acute toxicity results in arthralgias, myalgias, hemorrhagic gastroenteritis, kidney failure, and seizures. Long-term exposure can lead to confusion, headaches, skin and nail changes, paresthesias, weakness, and an increased cancer risk. Peripheral neuropathy can persist even after treatment.

Copper poisoning can occur in the context of *Wilson disease*, which is also known as *progressive hepatolenticular degeneration*. It is an autosomal recessive disease localized to mutations on chromosome 13, and it involves a deficiency of the copper-transporting protein ceruloplasmin. This deficiency leads to copper deposits in tissues throughout the body, especially the liver, brain (specifically, the lenticular formation comprised of the globus pallidus and putamen), kidney, and corneas (manifested as corneal Kayser–Fleischer rings). Wilson disease can develop either in childhood or later in life depending on the degree of mutation, but, without early diagnosis and treatment, the condition is slowly progressive until the individual's eventual death within 6 months to 5 years. It typically begins with hepatic dysfunction and progresses to include neurologic impairment with ataxia, rigidity, tremor, and dysarthria in 40% of patients by the second or third decade. Without treatment, as many as 25% of patients develop a dementia syndrome that includes behavior, mood, and psychotic disturbances.

The diagnosis of Wilson disease is made based on the clinical symptoms, liver biopsy, and laboratory tests showing low serum ceruloplasmin and copper levels and increased 24-hour urinary copper levels. If treatment begins early, the symptoms can be reversed and controlled with anticopper therapy, including the copper-chelating agents penicillamine and trientine and copper-depleting agents, such as zinc and tetrathiomolybdate. Improvement may take several months, and a recovery to baseline depends on the extent of symptoms.

Toxic exposure to *carbon monoxide* is one of the most common causes of poisoning in the United States, typically resulting from prolonged accidental exposure to excessive fumes from vehicles or home heating devices without adequate ventilation. Carbon monoxide poisoning is also seen in suicide attempts, in which intentional exposure to vehicle exhaust occurs in a closed space. Individuals who survive carbon monoxide poisoning usually make a full recovery, although a significant percentage may develop sequelae, including cognitive impairment, extrapyramidal symptoms, and other focal neurologic symptoms. A less common gas causing poisoning involves *carbon disulfide*, which is used in the manufacture of rayon and as a grain fumigant. Long-term exposure has been associated with behavioral and cognitive disturbances, ataxia, peripheral neuropathy, and parkinsonism.

Dementia Caused by Vitamin Deficiencies

Vitamin deficiencies in older individuals have many causes, including a lack of income to buy food, physical disability that limits their ability to purchase and/or prepare food, poor appetite, lack of education, unusual diets, eating disorders, alcoholism, apathy, dementia, dental problems, dysphagia, gastrointestinal disease, and malabsorption syndromes. Deficiencies of several key vitamins including vitamin B_{12} (cobalamin), folate, niacin (vitamin B_3), and thiamine (vitamin B_1) have been associated with various symptoms of cognitive impairment, apathy, mood disturbances, psychosis, and peripheral neuropathies. These conditions are less commonly encountered in Western countries because of the generally adequate nutrition and vitamin supplementation of many food products. A routine dementia workup should always include attention to the individual's typical diet; medical conditions and any medications that may affect his or her eating, digestion, and appetite; and the social and financial resources required to maintain adequate nutrition. Vitamin supplementation is an important part of dementia care.

Vitamin B_{12} (cobalamin) deficiency, a relatively common vitamin deficiency, is seen in 5% to 15% of older adults. The vitamin B_{12} supply depends on both the oral intake and the presence of a binding agent known as intrinsic factor that is produced by parietal cells in the stomach. Vitamin B_{12} deficiency has commonly been associated with the autoimmune disorder *pernicious anemia*, in which these cells have atrophied. Other risk factors for vitamin B_{12} deficiency include strict vegetarian diets, gastric resection or bypass surgery, malabsorption syndromes (e.g., celiac disease), inflammatory bowel disease, *Helicobacter pylori* infection, and the use of proton pump inhibitors. Symptoms of vitamin B_{12} deficiency include confusion, peripheral neuropathy (e.g., paresthesias, loss of vibratory and position sense), and macrocytic (or megaloblastic) anemia. A more severe condition associated with vitamin B_{12} deficiency is *subacute combined degeneration*, a demyelinating disorder associated with peripheral neuropathy, depression, and dementia.

Levels of vitamin B_{12} below 200 pg per mL are regarded as low, while levels between 200 and 350 pg per mL are considered borderline. A complete assessment may also include a search for elevations of the vitamin B_{12} metabolites methylmalonic acid and homocysteine, especially when the vitamin B_{12} level is low normal. Physicians should obtain a Schilling test when malabsorption is suspected. Although several different protocols are used, treatment usually involves the administration of 1,000 μg of vitamin B_{12} intramuscularly every month or an oral dose of 100 μg daily. The repletion of the levels may reverse some of the neurologic manifestations of a deficiency, but it may not improve the symptoms of dementia.

Folate deficiency is associated with macrocytic anemia and elevated homocysteine levels. Although folate is present in many foods, it is significantly degraded by cooking and canning. Psychiatric conditions associated with prolonged folate deficiency include depression and a dementia syndrome similar to that seen in vitamin B_{12} deficiency. Folate and vitamin B_{12} deficiency have also been associated with increased rates of AD, which are possibly due to the elevated homocysteine levels.

Niacin deficiency, also called pellagra, is rarely seen in developed countries because of their niacin-enriched bread products. Symptoms of niacin deficiency include diarrhea, dermatitis, and dementia. Associated psychiatric symptoms include depression and psychosis, while frontal release signs and parkinsonism constitute other neurologic symptoms.

Thiamine deficiency, also called beri beri, is rare; however, when it does occur, it is seen in association with Wernicke–Korsakoff syndrome. This state is seen classically in alcoholics with minimal nutritional intake other than alcohol.

DEMENTIA ASSOCIATED WITH INFECTIOUS DISEASES

Historically, infectious diseases have represented a significant cause of dementia; epidemics of neurosyphilis date back to the 16th century, and encephalitis lethargica affected millions of individuals in the decade that followed World War I. The advent of antibiotics in the 1940s virtually eliminated neurosyphilis, and the further development of antimicrobial, antifungal and, more recently, antiviral agents has blunted the potential impact of other infectious diseases. These medical developments have also contributed greatly to longer life spans, meaning that most individuals in developed countries live to the stages of life at highest risk of both AD and VaD. Consequently, the surge in prevalence of these dementia types in the past 50 years has eclipsed that of dementia caused by infectious sources. Unfortunately, the incidence of infectious dementias has been increasing as a result of the human immunodeficiency virus (HIV) pandemic and associated opportunistic infection sources.

Acute infection of the CNS can result in either a meningitis or an encephalitis characterized by fever, meningeal signs (headache, stiff neck, photophobia), mental status changes consistent with delirium (see Chapter 12 for more details), focal neurologic signs, and seizures. These emergent states require rapid medical intervention, but, even with aggressive treatment, they can sometimes lead to permanent neurologic symptoms, dementia, or death. Immunocompromised, older, and medically ill individuals are at greatest risk of developing encephalitis and its sequelae. Chronic infections of the CNS present more insidiously, and they may produce a dementia in which no clear evidence of the underlying source is found. Brain damage from infections can result from several of the following mechanisms: (a) the direct toxic effects of the pathogen and its products, (b) inflammatory responses, (c) opportunistic and secondary infections, and (d) immune-mediated postinfectious encephalitic states.

 TIP

Several clues in the dementia workup that may suggest an underlying infectious encephalitis include a recent viral or other unexplained illness or rash, seasonal or geographic proximity to epidemic or endemic illnesses (e.g., overseas travel), an acute onset of symptoms, seizures, extrapyramidal symptoms, and HIV infection. A thorough physical examination may reveal unrecognized sites of infections that can seed the CNS, such as tooth abscesses, cardiac valvular vegetations, and sinus infections. Neuroimaging may reveal occult abscesses in the CNS.

Infectious pathogens that can cause encephalitis and subsequent dementia include bacteria, viruses, spirochetes, fungi, and parasites. Also included in this category are the infectious proteinaceous particles, or *prions*, that cause the transmissible spongiform encephalopathies. Common infectious sources are summarized in Table 11.3. The requisite laboratory tests include a complete blood count, blood cultures, and an analysis of CSF. In viral encephalitis, CSF analysis typically shows a mild lymphocytosis with normal glucose and increased protein levels. In most cases of presumed viral illness, however, the source is never isolated, even with serologic investigation. CSF analysis in bacterial and fungal infections of the CNS is usually more revealing, with findings of gross lymphocytosis and elevated protein levels. CSF culture and staining can isolate bacteria and most fungi, but serologic studies, including

TABLE 11.3. Infectious Sources of Encephalitis and Dementia

Bacterial meningoencephalitides and abscesses
  Streptococcus pneumoniae, Neisseria meningitides, Listeria monocytogenes, Haemophilus influenzae Type b, *Mycoplasma pneumonia, Mycobacterium tuberculosis, Legionella pneumophila* (Legionnaire disease), *Rochalimaea henselae* (catscratch disease), brucellosis, *Tropheryma whippelii* (Whipple disease)

Viral encephalitides
  Human immunodeficiency virus 1; herpes simplex virus, types 1 and 2; Epstein–Barr virus; cytomegalovirus; mumps; influenza; coxsackie; rabies; flaviviruses (West Nile virus, yellow fever, dengue fever); arboviruses (St. Louis encephalitis, western and eastern equine encephalitis); papovavirus (JC virus)

Spirochetal encephalopathies
  Neurosyphilis (*Treponema pallidum*), Lyme disease (*Borrelia burgdorferi*)

Fungal meningitis and brain abscesses
  Cryptococcus, Coccidioides, Histoplasma, Aspergillus, Candida, Blastomyces, Actinomyces, Mucor, Sporothrix

Parasitic diseases and brain abscesses
  Rickettsial diseases (Q fever, typhus, Rocky Mountain spotted fever), toxoplasmosis, cysticercosis, amebic meningoencephalitis, malaria (*Plasmodium falciparum* and others), trypanosomiasis, trichinosis, strongyloidiasis, visceral larva migrans, schistosomiasis

Prion diseases
  Creutzfeldt–Jakob disease, variant Creutzfeldt–Jakob disease, kuru, Gertsmann–Sträussler–Scheinker syndrome, fatal familiar insomnia

Postinfectious dementias
  Subacute sclerosing panencephalitis (measles sequelae), encephalitis lethargica

immunologic markers, are needed for spirochetes and some fungi. Brain scans are typically normal in acute meningoencephalitis, but, in chronic infections, scans may demonstrate abscesses or focal neuronal loss or demyelination, especially in the basal ganglia. Electroencephalography (EEG) may demonstrate diffuse slowing with abnormal frontal and temporal rhythms across all types of infections.

Bacterial infections of the CNS are uncommon causes of dementia by their very nature; they are usually emergent, resulting rapidly in either recovery or death. However, undiagnosed bacterial brain abscesses and postinfectious processes may cause cognitive and behavioral disturbances, as well as seizures and other neurologic symptoms. The aggressive use of intravenous antibiotics is curative in many cases of acute bacterial encephalitis and in most cases of subacute or chronic infections. The most common causes of bacterial encephalitis in older individuals include *Streptococcus pneumoniae*, *Neisseria meningitides*, *Listeria monocytogenes*, and *Haemophilus influenzae* Type b. Other bacterial sources are listed in Table 11.3.

Viral infections are the most common cause of both acute and chronic encephalitis, with HIV representing the source of the most cases. The next most commonly reported viral sources include herpes simplex, influenza, measles, and Epstein–Barr virus. *Herpes simplex encephalitis* presents as an acute viral syndrome, and more than half of all cases occur in the elderly. The infection has a predilection for the mediotemporal and orbitofrontal cortices, and it is associated with frontal lobe symptoms. Dementia that is characterized by amnesia and aphasia is a possible postinfectious consequence. Damage to the mediotemporal lobes may result in Klüver–Bucy syndrome (see Chapter 10 for a complete discussion). Aggressive antiviral treatment is critical to decreasing the morbidity and mortality associated with many viral encephalitides.

Progressive multifocal leukoencephalopathy is a cerebral demyelinating disorder that results from infection with the JC virus, a ubiquitous human papovavirus. The virus apparently leaves its dormant state and begins active replication in susceptible individuals who are elderly, who have a hematologic cancer, or who are otherwise immunocompromised, including as many as 5% of patients with acquired immunodeficiency syndrome (AIDS). The clinical symptoms include a rapid onset of dementia, personality changes, and focal neurologic symptoms, including hemiparesis progressing to quadriparesis, aphasia, ataxia, visual disturbances, and dysarthria. Brain imaging reveals demyelinating lesions of various sizes. Death occurs within 3 to 6 months, although the use of antiretroviral therapy has led to variable outcomes in patients with AIDS.

Several rare dementing conditions, which are believed to represent chronic infection or an immune-mediated postinfectious condition, occur months to years after an acute viral infectious episode. *Subacute sclerosing panencephalitis* can occur in children 6 to 8 years after a bout of measles; it involves severe neurologic impairment and dementia that usually culminates in death within 1 to 3 years. It is rarely seen today because of the use of the measles vaccine. *Encephalitis lethargica*, which is also known as von Economo disease and sleeping sickness, affected nearly five million people in the decade after the influenza pandemic of 1917, but it has rarely been seen since 1930. This acute cortical and subcortical syndrome was characterized by profound lethargy ("sleeping"), ophthalmoplegia, parkinsonism, psychosis, and a fatal encephalitis in 20% to 30% of patients. Recovery from the acute syndrome was followed by the development of a parkinsonian syndrome months to years later and an ensuing subcortical dementia.

Spirochetes are motile microorganisms that cause CNS infections, including syphilis caused by *Treponema pallidum*, Lyme disease caused by *Borrelia burgdorferi*, and leptospirosis caused by *Leptospira interrogans*. Both syphilis and Lyme disease are described in detail in the next section.

Fungal CNS infections associated with encephalitis have become more common in the past 20 years as opportunistic infections occurring in the setting of HIV infection and other immunocompromised states. The range of fungal culprits includes *Cryptococcus*, *Coccidioides*, *Histoplasma*, *Aspergillus*, *Candida*, *Blastomyces*, *Actinomyces*, *Mucor*, and *Sporothrix* organisms. Fungal meningitis generally develops insidiously over weeks to months, producing classic meningeal signs. The complications can include cranial neuropathies, strokes, brain abscesses, and hydrocephalus. A diagnosis is usually made on the basis of CSF staining, cultures, or fungal antigen titers. Traditionally, antifungal treatment relied on intravenous or even intrathecal amphotericin B (Fungizone) with its associated toxicity, but several newer and less toxic triazole antifungal agents are now available for use. Cryptococcal meningitis, the most common fungal CNS infection, can produce focal neurologic symptoms and delirium, as well as a dementia with waxing and waning symptoms over months to years. The overall mortality rate approaches 40%.

CLINICAL VIGNETTE

Mr. Crown, a 38-year-old, HIV-positive man, had a several-week history of evolving headache, poor concentration, apathy, and memory impairment. He was diagnosed with HIV-1–associated dementia (HAD). The symptoms persisted despite adjustments in his antiretroviral regimen. Eventually, a spinal tap was performed, and the CSF analysis revealed cryptococcal meningitis. Treatment with amphotericin B led to a complete resolution of symptoms. Thus, a presumed case of HAD turned out to be a treatable opportunistic CNS infection.

Parasitic infections of the CNS are rare, but, like fungal infections, they are now seen more commonly in the setting of HIV infection and other immunocompromised states. These infections include organisms such as rickettsias (intracellular bacterial parasites), protozoa, and worms (cestodes, nematodes, and trematodes). Several other parasitic diseases are listed in Table 11.3. CNS involvement by each of these parasites can include meningoencephalitis, cerebral cysts, seizures, and hydrocephalus.

Human Immunodeficiency Virus Dementia

Infection with HIV is associated with direct viral damage to the CNS, which, in turn, leads to increasing degrees of neuropsychiatric impairment. Fifteen percent to 30% of HIV-infected individuals are estimated to demonstrate mild neuropsychologic impairment despite being otherwise asymptomatic. More significant impairment may constitute a diagnosis of HIV-associated minor cognitive disorder, which is characterized by the presence of all four of the following criteria as established by the American Academy of Neurology: (a) cognitive, motor, and behavioral abnormalities verified by the history and neuropsychologic tests; (b) mild impairment of work or the activities of daily living; (c) the symptoms do not meet the criteria for HIV dementia or HIV myelopathy; and (d) no other etiology is present.

More severe neuropsychologic impairment may represent a subcortical dementia termed HAD. Other names that have been used for this condition include HIV encephalopathy and AIDS dementia complex. According to the American Academy of Neurology, HAD is defined by the following:

1. Impairment in at least two of the following cognitive abilities for at least 1 month: attention and/or concentration,

abstraction and/or reasoning, visuospatial skills, memory learning, and language;
2. Decline in at least one of the following: motor function or performance, motivation or emotional control, or social behavior;
3. The impairment is not caused by delirium or any other disorder

The diagnosis of HAD is based on clinical symptoms because no specific diagnostic laboratory tests or radiographic findings have been identified. HAD may be seen as an initial manifestation of AIDS in nearly 20% of older patients. Previously, 15% to 20% of all AIDS patients developed HAD, but its prevalence has decreased to less than half of that because of the widespread use of combination antiretroviral therapies, which themselves can sometimes be a cause of transitory cognitive impairment or confusion.

The presence of HAD has been associated with increased mortality, and its identification should prompt aggressive management. In addition to antiretroviral therapy, psychostimulants such as methylphenidate (Ritalin) have been used with some success to treat the cognitive slowing and lethargy associated with HAD.

Neurosyphilis

Syphilis is a communicable disease caused by the spirochete *T. pallidum*, a spiral-shaped motile microorganism. It is primarily transmitted via the skin and mucous membranes during sexual contact, but it can also be spread by blood transfusions and perinatal contact. Syphilis involves several stages.

Primary syphilis: development of a chancre at the site of infection within several weeks with spontaneous resolution. The systemic spread is usually occult at this point.

Secondary syphilis: development of a red maculopapular rash on the body and condylomatous papules in the anogenital and axillary regions 2 to 10 weeks after primary syphilis, followed by spontaneous resolution. Thirty percent of infected individuals have no further manifestations after the primary or secondary stages, and another 30% have latent disease.

Tertiary syphilis: thirty percent of the infected individuals reach this stage years to decades after the primary infection, resulting in one or more of the following: granulomatous lesions in the skin, bones, and liver; cardiac and ophthalmologic problems; and CNS infection or neuro-syphilis.

Neurosyphilis is characterized by meningeal inflammation, frontal and temporal lobe demyelination, and cortical atrophy. The two major forms include *tabes dorsalis* and *general paresis*. The common symptoms of tabes dorsalis include peripheral neuropathy that is accompanied by pain in the extremities, ataxia, and incontinence. General paresis is characterized by the following:

- Progressive dementia with memory disturbances, disorientation, poor attention;
- Frontal lobe symptoms, such as personality change, apathy, and poor judgment;
- Psychosis in 10% to 20% of individuals, with hallucinations and paranoid or grandiose delusions;
- Mood disturbances, with mania being more common than depression;
- Neurologic symptoms, such as dysarthria, tremors, unsteady gait and ataxia, cranial neuropathies, loss of tone and reflexes, incontinence, pseudobulbar palsy, paralysis, and seizures.

Syphilis may be suspected based on clinical symptoms, but arriving at a definitive diagnosis relies on either nontreponemal antigenic tests (VDRL [Venereal Disease Research Laboratories] or rapid plasma reagin [commonly seen as RPR]) or treponemal detection (fluorescent treponemal antibody absorption test [commonly known as FTA-ABS]). The standard treatment for primary or secondary stage syphilis is 2.4 million U penicillin G intramuscularly. Tertiary syphilis, or neurosyphilis, requires the administration of intravenous penicillin. The symptoms of neurosyphilis can be reversed to variable degrees with successful treatment.

⬣ KEY POINT

Testing for syphilis with a rapid plasma reagin or VDRL test has always been a routine part of dementia workups, even though the infection has become quite uncommon. Even when syphilis does occur, seeing a case that has progressed to the tertiary stage is rare. Recent outbreaks of syphilis, however, should prompt all clinicians to include syphilis in the differential diagnosis, especially in individuals with known HIV infection or HIV risk factors.

Lyme Disease

Lyme disease is a tick-transmitted disease in humans that is caused by the spirochete *B. burgdorferi*. The disease is the most common vector-borne illness in the United States, and it has been associated with neurologic and psychiatric symptoms in nearly 40% of infected individuals. Although Lyme disease had been clinically described for decades, it was first identified and classified serologically after an outbreak of arthritis in a group of infected children in Lyme, Connecticut, in 1977. The initial stage of Lyme disease is a localized, target-shaped rash, called erythema migrans, at the site of a tick bite; its appearance is sometimes associated with the subsequent development of flulike symptoms. Early disseminated infection may then occur acutely days to weeks after infection or as a later stage months or years later; it is characterized by fever, fatigue, headache, migrating joint and tendon pain, and lymphadenopathy. CNS involvement may occur as cranial or peripheral neuropathies and a meningoencephalitis. Lyme encephalopathy or dementia that is characterized by mild to severe impairment in short-term memory, bradyphrenia, word-finding and reading difficulties, visuospatial impairment, and emotional lability can be seen in late-stage disease. Depression, which may serve to worsen the cognitive deficits, has also been linked with Lyme disease.

 TIP

When conducting a dementia workup, always inquire about tick bites or exposure to wooded areas endemic to ticks and Lyme disease. The standard blood test is a Lyme titer, which may give a false negative result in the first month after infection. In cases with a negative titer but a high index of suspicion, conducting an enzyme-linked immunosorbent assay or Western blot test may be necessary. In addition to serum titers, an analysis of the CSF should be considered when neurologic symptoms are present. The treatment of choice for Lyme disease is antibiotic therapy; with therapy, the prognosis is generally good for all symptoms.

Creuzfeldt–Jakob Disease

Creutzfeldt–Jakob disease (CJD) is one of several dementing illnesses that are believed to be caused by *proteinaceous infec-*

tious particles or *prions*. These illnesses are also called *prion diseases* because of their etiology and *transmissible spongiform encephalopathies* based on their pathology. All prion diseases are rapidly progressive neurodegenerative disorders that can affect both animals and humans and that share several common features, including the following: (a) they cause spongiform degeneration of the brain, (b) they are transmittable by prion-infected tissue, and (c) a long latency exists between the exposure and the appearance of symptoms. Apparently, only susceptible individuals develop symptoms. Known prion diseases in animals include scrapie in sheep, chronic wasting disease in deer, and bovine spongiform encephalopathy (BSE), also known as mad cow disease, in cattle. Chronic wasting disease has been spreading among the United States deer populations in the past few years, which has prompted the wholesale elimination of regional populations during extended deer hunting seasons. The increased presence of chronic wasting disease has also increased the anxiety regarding the safety of ingesting wild venison. Human prion diseases include kuru, CJD, variant CJD, Gerstmann–Straüssler–Scheinker syndrome, and fatal familial insomnia.

CJD, a rare form of dementia, is seen sporadically in individuals between the ages of 50 and 70 years. Between 5% and 15% of all cases are familial, which suggests that a genetic susceptibility to prion infection exists. Cases of CJD have also been seen in individuals exposed to infected brain tissue, such as may occur with the use of inadequately sterilized surgical instruments or the administration of growth hormone made from infected pituitary glands. A similar mode of transmission is seen with the prion disease kuru, which is found among members of one particular New Guinea tribe that practiced cannibalism of the brain tissue as part of their burial rites. The concept of infectious proteinaceous particles was proposed by Dr. Stanley Prusiner in 1982 and was greeted with much controversy. However, the existence and infectious nature of prions have come to be recognized in the decades since. Based on reviews of the methods of transmission, prions are clearly resistant to some methods of sterilization, such as boiling, formalin, and ultraviolet light, and the use of either bleach or pressure autoclaving is required.

From the appearance of the initial symptoms of CJD, the affected individual enters a rapidly progressive decline, followed by death, a clinical picture that takes, on average, 6 to 12 months. Early symptoms may include fatigue, insomnia, and anorexia, with a progression to dementia that is associated with behavioral disturbances and myoclonus. Depression and psychosis are seen in approximately 10% of cases, and detailed delusions and hallucinations may occur. The T2-weighted images from an MRI of the brain may show basal ganglia hyperintensity. The EEG shows periodic bursts of characteristic bifrontal sharp waves or triphasic waves that are set against a slowed background rhythm. The 14-3-3 protein, a biomarker associated with CJD, is found in the CSF.

Many of the persistent questions regarding the etiology of prion diseases came to the forefront during the epidemic of BSE in the United Kingdom in the late 1980s and early 1990s. At its peak, nearly 40,000 cases of BSE occurred, necessitating the mass slaughter and cremation of a large portion of the United Kingdom's cattle herd to stop the spread of the disease. The BSE epidemic was believed to have been caused by cows that were given feed containing infected neural tissue from other animals. After the BSE epidemic, nearly 100 cases of spongiform dementias have been seen in humans, presumably due to the consumption of meat products that contained infected neural tissue from cows with BSE. This new dementia was labeled variant CJD (vCJD).

Unlike CJD, vCJD strikes young individuals after an incubation period of approximately 6 years from the ingestion of tainted meat. Early manifestations of vCJD usually include psychiatric disturbances, such as personality changes, social withdrawal, depression, anxiety, and psychosis with complex delusions and hallucinations. Other symptoms include insomnia, excessive somnolence during the day, and anorexia, which then progress to include neurologic symptoms, such as myoclonus; ataxia; and pain and paresthesias in the extremities, head, and neck. Progressive dementia results in a mute, rigid state, with death occurring after an average course of 14 months. Although vCJD is presumed to result from contact with tissue from cattle with BSE, the exact method of transmission has not been confirmed because knowing with certainty whether someone had contact with such products is impossible. In addition, the sporadic nature of vCJD in the thousands of individuals who likely ate the same meat products raises questions about why some younger individuals were disproportionately affected. Ongoing research is investigating the role of a human prion protein gene and whether mutations might confer a genetic susceptibility to developing symptoms.

In addition to kuru, two other potential human prion diseases are Gerstmann–Straüssler–Scheinker syndrome and fatal familial insomnia. Both Gerstmann–Straüssler–Scheinker syndrome and fatal familial insomnia are rare disorders that strike middle-age adults; they are associated with genetic mutations in the prion protein gene. Gerstmann–Straüssler–Scheinker syndrome is an autosomal dominant disorder that is characterized by dementia with pyramidal, extrapyramidal, and cerebellar symptoms, whereas fatal familial insomnia is a rapidly progressive disease of thalamic nuclei that is characterized by multiple neurologic disturbances, a frontal lobe type of dementia, insomnia, and dysautonomia.

DEMENTIA CAUSED BY ORGAN FAILURE

More than 300,000 individuals in the United States have been diagnosed with chronic renal failure, and two-thirds are receiving hemodialysis. Chronic renal failure can cause a state of impaired cognitive functioning that is known as *uremic encephalopathy*. This state is best characterized as a form of delirium rather than as dementia. The early symptoms of headache, weakness, poor concentration, apathy, and irritability can progress to a more pronounced state of confusion, memory impairment, psychosis, agitation, and insomnia. The focal neurologic symptoms include tremor, asterixis, and a polyneuropathy seen in the majority of patients that involves painful sensations in the extremities. Later symptoms in untreated patients include myoclonus and seizures. The characteristic EEG findings in uremic encephalopathy occur at blood urea nitrogen levels greater than 60 mg per dL, and they include progressive slowing and disorganization of the background rhythm, with paroxysmal, bilateral bursts of slower waves. Improvement in the symptoms is slow, but they usually completely resolve with hemodialysis or renal transplant. Patients on dialysis once ran the risk of a fatal condition known as "dialysis dementia," which was attributed to aluminum poisoning from the dialysate solutions; it was characterized by cognitive decline, frontal lobe symptoms, and severe neurologic symptoms. A reduction in aluminum exposure has all but eliminated this disorder in dialysis patients.

Hepatic failure can cause an encephalopathy similar to uremia that is characterized by confusion, asterixis, ataxia, hyperreflexia, mood disturbances, and psychosis. Both neuropsychologic and positron emission tomography studies suggest the presence of predominantly bifrontal and biparietal impairment in hepatic encephalopathy, including declines in executive dysfunction and fine motor skills. The most common causes in adults and the elderly are alcohol-induced cirrhosis and chronic infectious hepatitis. The characteristic EEG findings include bilateral, frontal bursts of 2-Hz triphasic waves set against a slowed and disorganized background rhythm. Hepatic encephalopathy is attributed to increased serum levels of ammonia and other neurotoxins. Treatment involves a reduction in the intake of dietary protein as a source of ammonia and the use of an intestinal binding agent, such as lactulose or neomycin, for ammonia.

DEMENTIA ASSOCIATED WITH ENDOCRINE DISEASE

Endocrine diseases, which represent some of the most common late-life medical disorders, are associated with significant morbidity, including the potential for dementia.

Diabetes mellitus is the most common endocrine disorder, with the adult-onset or type II form affecting 20% of individuals older than the age of 80. The chronic hyperglycemia of diabetes mellitus causes both microvascular and macrovascular damage throughout the body, resulting in a significantly increased risk of peripheral vascular disease, myocardial infarction, and stroke. Not surprisingly, diabetes mellitus is found in nearly 50% of individuals with VaD, and it has been shown to nearly double the risk of both AD and VaD. Chronic episodes of hypoglycemia can also cause cognitive impairment, including memory impairment and behavioral disturbances.

Hypothyroidism, the second most common endocrine disease after diabetes mellitus, is characterized by a variety of neuropsychiatric symptoms, including lethargy, depression, apathy, slowed thinking (bradyphrenia), and dementia. However, improved surveillance by physicians has significantly reduced the risk of active disease reaching that point. The mood disturbances and mild cognitive impairment usually improve with treatment, but they can persist in as many as 10% of patients.

Hyperparathyroidism causes the excessive production of parathyroid hormone, which can result in hypercalcemia with resultant bone resorption and an increased risk of fracture, urinary calculi, gastrointestinal disturbances, and peptic ulcer disease. The most common cause of hyperparathyroidism is a parathyroid adenoma. The neuropsychiatric symptoms of this condition include depression in approximately 66% of patients; impaired memory in 25%; paranoid psychosis in 10%; and agitation, confusion, delirium, and personality changes, such as apathy. Mental status changes can also result from the associated metabolic disturbances, including hypophosphatemia, hypokalemia, and hypomagnesemia. The treatment can involve surgical resection of the adenoma or medication to reduce calcium levels. Hypocalcemia can also lead to confusion, cognitive impairment, and personality changes.

Cushing syndrome is associated with *hypercortisolemia*, and it results from adrenocortical hyperfunction. The most common cause of Cushing syndrome is excess production of adrenocorticotropic hormone in the anterior pituitary gland (Cushing disease), but adrenocortical hyperplasia can also be a cause. Hypercortisolemia can lead to numerous neuropsychiatric symptoms, including memory impairment, poor concentration and attention, bradyphrenia, impaired abstract thinking, and depression. *Addison disease*, or adrenocortical insufficiency, can also produce a slowly progressive dementia that is characterized by memory impairment, bradyphrenia, depression, and psychosis. Mental status changes in both Cushing syndrome and Addison disease can be reversed with the institution of the appropriate treatment.

DEMENTIA ASSOCIATED WITH CHRONIC NEUROLOGIC DISEASE

Regardless of the cause, a common pathologic end point in many cases of dementia is demyelination. Demyelinating disorders are characterized by the progressive loss of the myelin sheath or physiologic insulation on neurons, which leads to slowing and the disruption of axonal transmission. Myriad causes exist for the various demyelinating disorders, and these disorders can occur at any age.

Multiple Sclerosis

Multiple sclerosis (MS) is the most common demyelinating disorder seen in adults. MS is an autoimmune disorder that produces multiple areas of focal white matter demyelination in the CNS. It typically presents in early adulthood, with fewer than 1% of cases seen after the age of 60. MS is more prevalent in women and in northern latitudes. The initial presentations of MS are extremely variable, ranging from obvious pathognomonic symptoms to subtle and fluctuating ones that elude diagnosis. Not uncommonly, an individual with confounding symptoms will receive incorrect diagnoses and no definitive treatment; eventually, he or she may be given psychiatric designations for years before the disorder clearly establishes itself. One of the reasons for this delay is that the pathologic hallmark of MS, multiple sclerotic white matter plaques in the CNS representing areas of demyelination, may not appear or may not be clearly visualized on MRI until the symptoms have been present for some time. MS may follow one of several courses, ranging from a relapsing and/or remitting pattern of symptoms to a slowly or rapidly progressive course. A slowly progressive course is more common in older patients.

Acute symptoms include fatigue in 75% of patients, impaired motor function, gait disturbances and ataxia, spastic weakness, incontinence, optic neuritis, gaze palsies, and paresthesias. Neuropsychiatric symptoms include sexual dysfunction, sleep disturbances, apathy, depression, euphoria, and mania. Eventually, cognitive impairment is seen in 30% to 50% of patients with MS; this has frontal-subcortical characteristics, including memory impairment, slowed information processing, and executive dysfunction. The memory impairment affects both verbal and nonverbal memory, and it can influence immediate, anterograde, secondary, and remote memory. Language function is usually preserved in MS. The cognitive impairment can evolve into a clear dementia in 20% to 30% of patients with MS. Increased plaque volume and corpus callosum degeneration are the best predictors of cognitive impairment. No cure is available for MS, but the treatment has evolved significantly over the past few decades. Steroids, adrenocorticotropic hormone, immunosuppressive agents, and interferon β-1b have all been used to reduce the frequency and intensity of symptomatic attacks. Unfortunately, most individuals have residual neurologic impairment that accumulates with repeated episodes over years to decades.

OTHER DEMYELINATING DISORDERS

Several other demyelinating disorders causing cognitive impairment or dementia result from inherited metabolic disorders. *Adrenoleukodystrophy* is an X-linked demyelinating disorder of the cerebral white matter that is caused by a deficiency of a peroxidase enzyme; this results in the excessive storage of very-long-chain fatty acids. Adrenoleukodystrophy usually manifests in childhood, but 3% of cases present in adulthood, some as late as the age of 60. The adult form is associated with dementia and neurologic symptoms, including ataxia; paraparesis; dysarthria; impaired visual fields, acuity, and ocular movements; and hearing loss. Psychiatric symptoms, such as depression, agitation, mood lability, and psychosis, are seen in 40% of adults with adrenoleukodystrophy. Treatment with a diet low in very-long-chain fatty acids may reverse the symptoms or at least prevent the progression of the disorder, depending on when in the course of the disease it is initiated.

Metachromatic leukodystrophy, an inherited autosomal recessive demyelinating disorder that is related to a deficiency of arylsulfatase A, may present across the lifespan, but it is generally encountered between 16 and 40 years of age. It is characterized by the insidious development of global cognitive impairment, frontal lobe symptoms, and psychosis.

Cerebrotendinous xanthomatosis is an autosomal recessive disorder that causes increased levels of cholestanol because of the impaired hepatic synthesis of bile salts. Multiple neurologic symptoms are found in addition to dementia; these include neuropathy, dysarthria, seizures, and cerebral and tendinous xanthomas. Treatment with chenodeoxycholic acid can reverse the symptoms.

Huntington Disease

Huntington disease is a progressive neurodegenerative genetic disease that is associated with a dyskinetic movement disorder, dementia, and psychiatric disturbances. It has been linked with mutations on chromosome 4, and it is transmitted in an autosomal dominant manner, meaning that at least 50% of all offspring will be affected. The key pathologic feature is atrophy of the striatum (caudate and putamen), followed by eventual cerebral atrophy and ventricular dilation. The clinical symptoms of Huntington disease typically begin in the late 30s to early 40s; they include changes in personality (e.g., apathy, impulsivity) and behavior, as well as slowly evolving involuntary dyskinetic movements. The initial fidgeting movements in the hands and extremities progress to more general dyskinetic movements, including chorea and athetosis. Gaze palsies, dysarthria, decreased coordination with an abnormal and unsteady gait, orolingual apraxias, and increasing rigidity and dystonias are some of the associated neurologic symptoms that develop. Psychiatric disturbances, including depression, mania, or psychosis, are seen in 10% to 40% of patients with Huntington disease.

The dementia associated with Huntington disease begins with memory deficits and progresses over the course of the disease to encompass more global impairment, including visuospatial impairment, apraxias, dyscalculia, language disturbances, and executive dysfunction. No effective treatment exists for Huntington disease, and it progresses over 15 to 20 years until eventual death. Antipsychotic medications have been used to treat the behavioral disturbances, psychosis, and dyskinetic movements.

DEMENTIA CAUSED BY INFLAMMATORY DISEASES

Several inflammatory diseases, including collagen vascular diseases and vasculitides, can cause dementia. The mechanism of cognitive impairment is typically the immune-mediated destruction of small blood vessels, leading to tissue microinfarcts throughout the body. In general, these diseases are rare, and dementia is the result of severe and long-standing illness. Consequently, most individuals who present for a dementia workup generally have a history of many other symptoms and often a specific diagnosis. However, in the absence of a diagnosis, the clinician should obtain an erythrocyte sedimentation rate, which is a nonspecific marker for systemic inflammation. Although more specific tests are indicated for various diagnoses, rheumatologic and/or neurologic consultation is advised when an inflammatory disease is suspected.

The systemic symptoms common to most inflammatory diseases are fever, weight loss, headache, arthritis, and skin lesions. CNS involvement is seen in one-third to two-thirds of the affected individuals; a range of symptoms is seen, including cranial neuropathies, delirium, dysarthria, ataxia, ocular movement disturbances, corticospinal tract signs (e.g., paresis, spasticity), seizures, strokelike attacks, and dementia. Dementia caused by inflammatory diseases usually involves the frontotemporal lobe, with memory and language impairment, executive dysfunction, personality changes (e.g., apathy, disinhibition), psychosis, and mood disturbances. The treatment varies with each disease, but, in general, corticosteroids, antiinflammatory agents, cytotoxic agents, and immunosuppressive therapy are used.

The main collagen vascular diseases causing dementia are Behçet syndrome, Sjögren syndrome, and systemic lupus erythematosus. Of the three, *systemic lupus erythematosus* is the most common, involving the CNS in as many as 75% of cases. Vasculitides that cause dementia include granulomatous angiitis, lymphomatoid granulomatosis, polyarteritis nodosa, and Wegener granulomatosis. Of these four, *granulomatous angiitis* is the only disease in which the symptoms are confined to the CNS. Encephalopathy is an initial symptom of granulomatous angiitis, and the disease has a relatively poor prognosis in most patients. Given its rarity and short course, it generally is not seen in dementia clinics. *Lymphomatoid granulomatosis*, an inflammatory condition involving T-cell lymphocytic infiltration of lungs, skin, and nervous system, is primarily associated with lymphoma and CNS involvement in 20% to 40% of patients. *Polyarteritis nodosa* is a necrotizing vasculitis that is commonly seen in middle-aged women. Severe cognitive impairment and psychiatric symptoms are observed in as many as 20% of the affected individuals. *Wegener granulomatosis* is a vasculitis with necrotizing granulomas that are usually confined to the lungs and kidney. However, it can produce CNS involvement, including vascular damage to the brain.

PSYCHIATRIC CONDITIONS ASSOCIATED WITH DEMENTIA

Assessment of Agitation and Psychosis

Essential Concepts
- Agitation and psychosis are two of the most common psychiatric problems associated with dementia.
- Medical and psychiatric disorders and environmental stresses are common causes of agitation and psychosis.
- Delirium is an important and potentially life-threatening cause of agitation and psychosis that must be distinguished from dementia.
- The rudiments of assessment attempt to describe the behavioral problems and then to identify antecedent triggers, concurrent conditions, and consequences.

All forms of dementia have a strong association with the psychiatric symptoms of agitation and psychosis. Agitation is seen in 60% to 80% of individuals with dementia at some point during the course of their illness, whereas psychosis is seen in 35% to 50%. In this chapter, the two entities are discussed together because they commonly present in concert. For example, an individual with paranoid psychosis often presents with agitation. Although these symptoms may be present early in the course of a dementia, their frequency and intensity usually peak during the moderate stages of the dementia and then begin to decline as they enter the more severe stages. Agitation and psychosis are particularly disruptive to the lives of the affected individuals and their caregivers, and, frequently, they give rise to excess disability; threats to both personal health and the safety of others; emergent medical visits; acute hospitalization; and, ultimately, long-term institutionalization. The early recognition and treatment of these symptoms can mitigate these consequences, however, thus reducing the stress to the patients and the burden on their caregivers. A secondary benefit comes in terms of the significant economic savings for medical, psychiatric, and institutional care.

CLINICAL VIGNETTE

Mrs. Drum was an 82-year-old woman with a 4-year history of moderate vascular dementia and a long-standing history of a paranoid personality. She lived with her daughter, son-in-law, and two young grandchildren. A home health aide visited weekly to help with bathing Mrs. Drum after her daughter began a part-time job. However, Mrs. Drum was suspicious of the aide, and she frequently refused care due to paranoid concerns that the aide was trying to hurt her. After noticing that the aide was pregnant, Mrs. Drum told her daughter that the aide must have had an affair with her son-in-law and that she was trying to break up the family. The daughter tried to dispel her mother's concerns, but she did not intervene further. A week later Mrs. Drum became acutely agitated when the aide visited, and she began screaming at her not to touch her and to leave her family alone. When the aide attempted to approach Mrs. Drum to calm her, she lunged at the aide with her walker, threatening to kill the baby. The aide fled the house in tears and lodged a complaint with the agency. Her daughter returned home to find several police cars in front of her home; they had come in response to a hysterical call to 911 that Mrs. Drum had made, saying that someone was trying to kill her. Mrs. Drum began screaming and swearing at her daughter and the police, accusing them of leaving her alone to be killed. The two young grandchildren were terrified of the scene, and they began crying hysterically. Mrs. Drum was taken to an emergency department for evaluation and was subsequently hospitalized on a geriatric psychiatry unit. Given the severity of her episode of psychosis and agitation, the family decided to admit Mrs. Drum to a nearby nursing home.

This case is not at all uncommon. Unfortunately, the family did not fully appreciate the risk of behavioral problems that could result when Mrs. Drum began reporting her paranoid delusions. Earlier intervention might have prevented this terrible episode. Because the severity of the episode was so upsetting to the family, Mrs. Drum's continued residence at their home was no longer safe or appropriate. She needed a more structured and secure environment.

WHAT IS AGITATION? WHAT IS PSYCHOSIS?

The term agitation is used throughout the chapter to describe a variety of inappropriate verbal, vocal, and/or motor behaviors that are seen in association with dementia, including the following:

- **Verbal or physical aggression, assaultiveness, or abuse:** yelling, screaming, cursing, insulting, threatening, hitting, pushing, grabbing, pinching, kicking, biting, spitting, throwing or destroying property, combativeness.
- **Repetitive or hyperactive verbalizations, vocalizations, or motor behaviors:** calling out of words, phrases, or sounds repeatedly; repeated requests or demands regardless of the response; odd or unusual repetitive mannerisms; intrusive wandering.
- **Disinhibited or inappropriate behaviors or verbalizations:** public disrobing or nudity; public masturbation; groping or fondling others; obscene comments; smearing feces; attempting to open or to enter unsafe areas, such as windows, stairwells, and traffic.

Psychosis is defined as a mental state that is out of touch with reality because of false beliefs, perceptions, or disorganization. Common manifestations include the following:

- **Delusions** (false, fixed ideas)
  - Paranoid type ("someone is trying to kill me")
  - Grandiose type ("I am leading a platoon of men to hunt terrorists")
  - Jealous type ("my wife is having an affair with other residents")
  - Misidentification ("that is not the nurse, that is my mother")
- **Hallucinations** (false sensory percepts): most often auditory or visual
- **Formal thought disorder** (distinct from cognitive impairment)
  - Disorganized thought process (e.g., loose associations)
  - Bizarre or unusual use of language (e.g., clanging) or mannerisms

Agitation is easier to detect because it is observable, whereas a diagnosis of psychosis often relies on patient reports, which can be confusing, unreliable, and reflective of nonpsychotic experiences. The latter point is especially valid when the clinician is trying to distinguish a formal thought disorder from the disturbances in thinking and language that define the dementia.

CAUSES OF AGITATION AND PSYCHOSIS

Agitation and psychosis are multidetermined phenomena, which means that several factors occur and interact simultaneously to trigger the problematic behaviors. The major causes include the following:

- Dementia itself;
- Medical illness;
- Delirium;
- Medications;
- Pain and/or physical discomfort;
- Psychiatric illness;
- Sleep problems;
- Stress (psychologic and environmental).

An individual with a dementia can manifest agitation or psychosis simply as a result of the underlying impairment in brain circuits or neurochemistry critical to the control and expression of behavior. In particular, agitation and impulsivity have been associated with frontal and temporal lobe hypometabolism, whereas psychosis has been associated with damage to the middle frontal cortex and temporal lobe. Agitation and psychosis have also been associated with excess dopaminergic activity and with deficient cholinergic and serotonergic activity. Psychopharmacologic strategies exploit these hypotheses. In general, all forms of dementia give rise to agitation and psychosis, although a preponderance of disinhibited behaviors are associated with frontotemporal dementias while hallucinations are generally associated with dementia with Lewy bodies.

Medical illness can trigger acute symptoms of agitation and psychosis, and it can complicate any preexisting symptoms. The clinician should bear in mind that the demented brain is especially vulnerable to metabolic changes that normally would not cause problems in the nondemented brain. The risk of compromised brain function is particularly high with any medical condition that impairs the flow of oxygen or

TABLE 12.1. **Medical Problems Commonly Associated with Agitation, Psychosis, and Delirium**

Infection
Acute renal, hepatic, or thyroid dysfunction
Sensory impairment or loss (blindness, deafness)
Metabolic disturbances
Acute neurologic events
Acute cardiac events
Acute pulmonary events
Occult malignancies (especially in the central nervous system)
Occult bone fracture
Postoperative state
Substance intoxication or withdrawal

blood to the brain, which usually results in a state of delirium. Medical conditions commonly associated with agitation, psychosis, and delirium are listed in Table 12.1.

 TIP

The mechanism by which infection and other illnesses cause behavioral problems or delirium is not always clear, and the clinical symptoms of underlying medical illness are not always obvious. The rule of thumb for evaluating acute behavioral changes is that one should always conduct a urinalysis and urine culture and that medical consultation should always be obtained. The first step is important because urinary tract infections are the most common cause of delirium in nursing home populations and, by extension, in older individuals with dementia. While the clinician is awaiting medical consultation, the vital signs, fingerstick glucose level, and oxygen saturation should be checked. Any medication changes occurring in the past few weeks should be reviewed, and the clinician should inquire about recent injuries, especially those involving head trauma.

WHAT IS DELIRIUM?

Delirium is defined as an acute, transient, reversible brain syndrome that is characterized by fluctuating disturbances of consciousness, attention, perception, cognition, and neuropsychiatric function (e.g., sleep, appetite, psychomotor activity). Clinicians sometimes fail to diagnose delirium because it fluctuates over time and it can be confused with preexisting symptoms of dementia. Table 12.2 lists some of the main features for distinguishing between dementia and delirium. Delirium is an especially dangerous condition because it typically lasts for weeks to months and it is associated with mortality rates as high as 40% in the first year. Although delirium is considered reversible, it can severely

TABLE 12.2. Dementia Versus Delirium: Clinical Differences

Clinical feature	Delirium	Dementia
Onset	Acute, over days to weeks	Insidious, over months to years
Course	Fluctuating symptoms	Stable but with progressive decline
Duration	Days to weeks or months	Years until inevitable death
Awareness	Reduced	Clear
Attention	Impaired— distractible	Usually normal for discrete tasks
Alertness	Fluctuates, often lethargic or hypervigilant	Usually normal
Orientation	Impaired	Impaired
Memory	Immediate and recent memories impaired	Recent and remote memories impaired
Perception	Hallucinations common	Intact
Thinking	Fragmented and disorganized with transient delusions	Impaired abstract thinking, vague content, agnosia
Language	Speech slow or rapid, often incoherent	Word-finding difficulty, aphasia
Psychomotor	Variable— hyperkinetic or hypokinetic	Apraxia as dementia progresses
Sleep–wake cycle	Disrupted or reversed	Reversed or fragmented

disrupt medical and rehabilitative recovery, it can unmask or even cause enduring cognitive impairment, and it can lead to long-standing functional decline.

Delirium always has a medical cause. The method by which medical problems trigger delirium is unclear, but one avenue may be through the disruption of cholinergic function. In individuals with dementia, the risk factors for delirium include advancing age, infection, fractures, malnutrition, low albumin levels, sensory deprivation, physical restraints, and bladder catheters. Other medical causes of delirium are listed in Table 12.1. In long-term care settings, urinary tract infections are the most common cause of delirium. Delirium is particularly common in postoperative states, and it is seen in 30% to 40% of older individuals after hip and other orthopedic surgeries due to factors such as anesthesia, dehydration, anemia, and narcotic analgesics. Medications, especially those with anticholinergic, narcotic, antihistaminic, and sedative effects, are often the cause of dementia. Commonly prescribed anticholinergic medications are listed in Table 3.2. Some individuals also show a particular sensitivity to steroids and some antibiotics. In some cases, the sudden discontinuation of a medication is more of a problem than the medication itself because of withdrawal symptoms. Medications that commonly cause withdrawal after extended use (i.e., months to years) include benzodiazepines, narcotics, stimulants, steroids, and selective serotonin reuptake inhibitors.

◈ KEY POINT

Remember that all tricyclic antidepressants (TCAs), especially amitriptyline (Elavil), imipramine (Tofranil), and doxepin (Sinequan), have strong anticholinergic effects. Peripherally, these can lead to dry mouth, blurred vision, constipation, and urinary retention. Centrally, these can lead to confusion and delirium. TCAs can also cause excess sedation, increased heart rate, and orthostasis, and they can slow cardiac conduction. If a TCA is absolutely indicated, nortriptyline and desipramine have the least anticholinergic properties of all the TCAs, although both must still be used with great caution. Heart rate and blood pressure should always be checked and documented, and an electrocardiogram should be performed before treatment and then at regular intervals during treatment.

CLINICAL VIGNETTE

Mrs. Axel was an 82-year-old woman with Alzheimer disease who lived in an assisted-living facility. She had a moderate degree of cognitive impairment, but she was oriented to her surroundings and she enjoyed numerous social relationships. Mrs. Axel had a history of atrial fibrillation and was taking digoxin and Coumadin. She developed urinary incontinence due to bladder spasms, so she was started on bethanecol. Her functioning was relatively stable until her physician started her on low-dose amitriptyline to treat her chronic pain symptoms. Shortly thereafter, observers noted that Mrs. Axel had become more confused. One evening she wandered out of the assisted-living facility and got lost in the neighborhood. Several hours later, police found a confused, frightened, and slightly dehydrated Mrs. Axel pounding on the door of an empty house.

Mrs. Axel was experiencing an episode of acute confusion or delirium due to the excessive anticholinergic load in her body, which compromised the already marginal cholinergic brain function that is associated with her diagnosis of Alzheimer disease. As Table 3.2 shows, many medications commonly prescribed to the elderly, including digoxin, Coumadin, and especially bethanecol, have anticholinergic properties. The addition of the strongly anticholinergic TCA was what overwhelmed Mrs. Axel's cholinergic functioning and precipitated the delirium.

Physical pain or discomfort associated with medical conditions, even that accompanying seemingly innocuous states, such as constipation, pruritus, or excess hunger or thirst, can precipitate both agitation and psychosis. Pain is an especially influential trigger in those individuals who cannot adequately communicate their discomfort because of aphasia or disorganized thinking. These individuals may act out their pain, often in a manner that does not give a clear indication of the true problem to caregivers. Identifying this underlying discomfort is crucial so that patients are not given medication to calm them while the true cause of their suffering is missed. When pain is suspected, a test dose of an analgesic, such as acetaminophen, may be warranted.

Psychiatric illness can cause and shape agitation and psychosis through the influence of comorbid symptoms or the rekindling of past disorders. The common psychiatric disorders that give rise to behavioral problems include depression, anxiety, mania (bipolar disorder), panic disorder, and posttraumatic stress disorder. The detection of psychiatric symptoms requires a consideration of how the effects of aging and dementia may obscure or change the way in which they present, compared with their presentation in younger individuals or those without dementia. For example, depression in dementia may manifest as pain or other somatic complaints, withdrawal, irritability, or preoccupations with deceased relatives, in addition to or in lieu of the standard symptoms (see Chapter 14). Mania might present as repetitive vocalizations, lack of sleep, and restless motor activity, while anxiety may present with excessive crying, moaning, or fearful yelling. In addition to the major psychiatric disorders, underlying personality disorders that are characterized by inflexible and maladaptive behavioral patterns can have profound influences on agitation and psychosis. Such individuals may exhibit even more flagrant and more difficult behaviors when they are confronted with the confusion, disability, and unfamiliar and frustrating situations that are associated with dementia.

CLINICAL VIGNETTE

Mrs. Major was a 92-year-old woman with vascular dementia who, before the onset of her disease, was a reasonably well-functioning individual with an obsessive-compulsive personality. As long as she had a strong memory and plenty of time and independence, she was able to structure her daily life according to her lifelong rules and schedules. However, memory loss, mild aphasia, and macular degeneration made keeping her papers organized and managing her finances increasingly difficult for her. Her son eventually took over these responsibilities, which caused her to complain to him and to berate him for supposed mismanagement that she could not fully describe or reconcile. Dining room staff members at her assisted-living facility complained that she was harassing them with obscene and verbally abusive language and repetitive requests for particular foods and manner of preparation.

Eventually, she was asked to leave the assisted-living facility because of her behaviors.

In Mrs. Major's case, age-related sensory loss and symptoms of dementia diminished her ability to engage in an obsessive-compulsive style, despite the persistence of her dysfunctional tendencies. The ensuing frustration led to new symptoms of agitation and psychosis as she attempted to express her exasperation and to maintain a sense of control over her life.

Sleep disorders comprise a subset of psychiatric disorders that are extremely common in dementia due to the disruptive effects of progressive brain damage on the normal sleep architecture. Individuals with dementia tend to have less efficient sleep because of increased nighttime arousals, a loss of rapid eye movement sleep, and the breakdown of the circadian rhythms that previously enabled them to maintain a normal sleep-wake cycle. Moreover, older individuals with dementia rarely receive comprehensive sleep evaluations; instead, they are often treated with increasing doses of sedative-hypnotics that then compound the problem. The result can be irritability, poor daytime function, and agitation. Sundowning is one type of agitation occurring in the early evening or nighttime, perhaps as a result of accumulated fatigue or the inability to recognize time cues.

Environmental stress is often a cause or, at the very least, a contributing factor to agitation and psychosis. Common environmental stresses include unfamiliar or uncomfortable surroundings (e.g., excess heat, cold, or noise), moves from familiar to unfamiliar settings (e.g., nursing home placement, room changes), and disruptive caregivers or roommates. Hearing and/or visual loss can limit an individual's ability to perceive and to adjust to the changes occurring around him or her. The sense of confusion and increased disorientation after moves can be so frightening and threatening to individuals with poor memory and insight that they strike out in what they perceive to be self-defense. This "fight-or-flight" response, which is hardwired into the human brain, remains intact well into the later stages of a progressive dementia. The individual's baseline personality characteristics—to the extent that the personality remains intact—partially determine the manner in which the patient with dementia copes with stress. Individuals with inflexible personality traits are particularly prone to stress-induced behavioral problems.

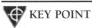 KEY POINT

One major stress for many individuals with dementia is living in an environment with excessive social and functional demands. When such individuals are unable to keep up with daily needs and they feel uncomfortable interacting in socially appropriate and competent ways with people without dementia, the result may be frustration, anger, anxiety, uncertainty, social with-drawal, or even disruptive behaviors in an attempt to cope with such an environment. Sometimes, the individuals themselves or their families force them into such situations because of pride, stubbornness, ignorance, or poor judgment. They are often motivated by a fear of nursing home placement.

ASSESSMENT OF AGITATION AND PSYCHOSIS

The assessment of agitation and psychosis involves the following two basic steps: (a) establishing a clear description of the problematic behaviors and (b) identifying their potential causes. A summary of the assessment process can be found on Pocket Card B.1 in Appendix B. The necessary information that should be obtained is summarized with the mnemonic ABCs:

Antecedents

- Is there anything occurring that seems to trigger the behaviors?
- Do they occur at a particular time of day?
- Are they associated with a particular person?
- Have any recent changes been made to the affected individual's schedule, location, or medications?

Behaviors

- What is reported as the problem by the patient and by caregivers?
- Have actual or threatened injuries to the patient or others occurred?
- Are the observed behaviors consistent with the reports? If not, how are they different?

- Are problematic behaviors new or recurrent?
- If they are recurrent, are they similar or different from past behaviors?
- Who is bothered by the behaviors (patient, staff, other residents)?

Concurrent/Comorbid Stresses

- Are concurrent environmental stresses that may be relevant present?
- Does the patient have comorbid medical or psychiatric disorders?

Consequences

- What results from the behaviors?
- Are they reinforced in any way?

 TIP

During an evaluation, keep in mind that most problematic behaviors are intermittent and often situational and that they likely will not present during a clinical interview. In addition, records and caregiver reports are not always accurate or reliable. You may hear different, and sometimes contradictory, descriptions from various staff members on a unit, or you may be told about a woman's terrible behavioral problems and then meet a "sweet little old lady" that you cannot imagine misbehaving. Caregivers may minimize or exaggerate their concerns; sometimes, discerning the truth is difficult because you do not know their reporting style. Do not rush to judgment; gather information from a variety of sources, corroborate these reports, and inquire about possible explanations. Careful investigation helps the clinician avoid unnecessary or misguided treatment.

Antecedent factors may include specific caregiving activities, individual contacts, and a time of day. For example, an individual with dementia and paranoia may react to being bathed or dressed as if he or she were being harmed. Such individuals may appear nervous and suspicious to their caregivers, and they may demonstrate overt paranoid ideation and physical resistance to care. The reasons behind these reactions may not be apparent or logical, but the association is important to notice. Taking note of the consequences of the behaviors is also essential. Do caregivers or staff react in such a manner as to reinforce the behaviors? Laughing at obscene comments or gestures or giving excessive attention to repetitive demands or aggressive movements may, in those patients with sufficient memory capacity, actually increase the frequency of the behavior.

With any potential behavioral problem, check to ensure that the complaints that are reported are consistent with what is actually taking place and that innocuous behaviors are not being misinterpreted or that, conversely, worrisome behaviors are not being dismissed.

CLINICAL VIGNETTE

Nurses reported that Mr. W. was acting in a sexually inappropriate way on the unit. A review of the chart indicated that he was seen walking down the hallway while exposing his genitals. Further discussion with staff members revealed that Mr. W. had severe dementia and that he did not know how to fasten his pants after using the bathroom. As a result, he frequently wandered into the hallway with his pants down, trying to get assistance.

In the case of Mr. W., a behavior was misinterpreted as representing sexual disinhibition, when it really represented confusion, apraxia, and an attempt to communicate nonverbally. This case illustrates how some behaviors can be considered "normal" in the context of dementia, instead of being labeled forms of agitation that warrant treatment. Examples of such "normal" behaviors in dementia include wandering, reaching out toward others, incoherent vocalizations, and unintentional incontinence or disrobing.

Psychotic symptoms can range from subtle to obvious, and they can easily be confused with nonpsychotic symptoms. For example, when a patient insists that he or she saw a deceased loved one, this can reflect an actual visual hallucination, a delusion of misidentification (i.e., the false, fixed belief that another person is the deceased loved one), or simply confusion associated with the dementia itself (e.g., an unfamiliar person is mistaken for a familiar one, perhaps because of similar physical characteristics or because the misidentified person's death was forgotten). Hallucinations can occur in all sensory modalities, but they are usually auditory or visual. Hallucinations reported by a person with dementia can be difficult to distinguish from confused descriptions of sensory input, images from dreams, and illusions (i.e., misinterpretations of sensory stimuli). The presence of psychotic symptoms should always prompt a search for medications that can induce them, especially in Parkinson disease or dementia with Lewy bodies.

WHO IS BEING TREATED?

Understanding who is most concerned about the behaviors and why they are is important. The goal, of course, is to treat the patient first and then attend to the stress felt by caregivers or institutional staff. A wandering or a hypervocal patient may not be in any personal distress, but he or she may be a significant annoyance to a caregiver or other residents or staff in a long-term care facility. Obviously, treating an individual for a problem that someone else is having is not ethical; however, ignoring the stress felt by caregivers, staff, or residents can have a negative effect on care by increasing the overall caregiver burden and/or acuity on a ward. The key is to determine whether the patient or other individuals are at any risk of harm due to injury, neglect, or an inability to provide care. If none of these risks exists, the caregivers and staff have the responsibility to provide a safe and appropriate environment for the behaviors and to seek the counsel of others to deal with their own stress rather than to impose it on the patient.

MEDICAL AND DELIRIUM WORKUP

A medical workup is always indicated for (a) suspicion of delirium, (b) sudden changes in behavior, and (c) treatment-resistant problems. For these acute changes, the obvious goal of this workup is to identify an etiology that can be treated to resolve the behavioral problems or delirium. The medical workup and the delirium workup are identical, and they should at least include the following:

- Physical and neurologic examinations;
- Laboratory tests: complete blood count, electrolytes, calcium, blood urea nitrogen/creatinine, relevant medication levels;

- Urinalysis (plus culture and sensitivity);
- Brief cognitive screen.

Depending on the patient's presentation, history, and test results, additional tests may be performed, including liver and thyroid function tests, a toxicology screen, bacterial cultures, cerebrospinal fluid analysis and culture, electrocardiography, brain computed tomography or magnetic resonance imaging, and other relevant radiographs.

When the clinician is uncertain about whether delirium is present, he or she should refer to Table 12.2 and should review the clinical differences between the presentations of dementia and delirium. In addition, several rating scales can help to identify delirium. One of the most widely used is the Delirium Rating Scale, a 10-item, clinician-rated scale that measures symptoms of delirium and tracks its progress. A shorter and more practical scale for use in the clinic or at the bedside is the Confusion Assessment Method Diagnostic Algorithm, which is found on Pocket Card B.2 in Appendix B. The Confusion Assessment Method Diagnostic Algorithm was designed for use in a hospital setting, but it can be applied in the clinic and nursing home as well.

BEHAVIORAL RATING SCALES

Numerous behavioral rating scales can be used to establish a quantitative baseline to assess the degree and scope of an individual's behavioral problems and to track his or her progress. For the average clinician, using these scales is not always practical during routine visits, but they can be quite valuable in formal dementia workups and they are essential in research. Some of these scales are the Behavior Pathology in Alzheimer's Disease Rating Scale, the Behavior Rating Scale for Dementia, the Brief Psychiatric Rating Scale, the Cohen–Mansfield Agitation Inventory, the Overt Aggression Scale, the Neuropsychiatric Inventory, and the Rating Scale for Aggressive Behavior in the Elderly.

Most of these scales require information from an informant. The Neuropsychiatric Inventory, or NPI, is the most extensive of the scales, and it has become quite popular in clinical drug trials. It examines the frequency and severity of behaviors in the following 12 symptom domains: agitation and aggression, disinhibition, apathy, dysphoria, euphoria, irritability and lability, disinhibition, delusions, hallucinations, sleep and appetite disturbances, and aberrant motor behavior. The Behavior Pathology in Alzheimer's Disease Rating Scale has also been extensively used in drug trials that focus on Alzheimer disease. The Cohen–Mansfield Agitation Inventory, or CMAI, focuses more on agitation and aggression; it is a staple of clinical trials that involve nursing home residents.

Treatment of Agitation and Psychosis

Essential Concepts
- The first step in the treatment of agitation and psychosis is to identify and to address the underlying causes. The second step is to implement an environmental or behavioral plan. When these two steps fail, the third step is to use appropriate psychopharmacologic treatment.
- The atypical antipsychotic medications are generally the most effective psychopharmacologic agents for both agitation and psychosis.
- Treatment failure requires a reassessment of the diagnosis, causes, and adequacy of pharmacotherapy. Trials of alternate pharmacologic agents, whether alone or in combination, are often warranted.
- Behavioral emergencies require that prompt attention is devoted to calming the individual; removing any triggers; and, when necessary, providing rapidly effective pharmacologic agents.

The assessment of agitation and psychosis, as described in Chapter 12, lays the basis for treatment. As the clinician begins to synthesize all of the available clinical information and to think about devising a direction for treatment, the following principles should be kept in mind.

Do not go it alone. A team approach is the best way of addressing agitation and psychosis. Team members may include physicians, psychologists, nurses, social workers, and other health care providers or support staff. Working together, the team can best identify the causes and can select the most appropriate and realistic target symptoms and interventions.

Recognize the power of environmental and behavioral interventions. Behavioral strategies do not need to be elaborate to be effective. For many individuals with dementia with agitation, a caring environment with adequate structure can sometimes be the most effective intervention. The clinician should not assume that an individual with severe dementia is oblivious to the environment or to his or her conduct, even when the patient is in the severe stages of dementia.

Be patient and allow time, effort, and creativity to work. Interventions do not always work quickly, and they may require numerous attempts and revisions to work. Be persistent. If one approach does not work, try another. Do not rely on the same approach for each patient.

PUTTING THE *TREAT* IN TREATMENT

One way to approach treatment for agitation and psychosis is summarized by the following mnemonic TREAT:

Target symptoms: define target symptoms.
Reversible causes: treat reversible causes.
Environment: optimize the environment and implement a behavior plan.
Agents: when necessary, select an appropriate psychopharmacologic agent.
Try again: if the improvement is insufficient, try again.

Each step is reviewed in detail in the following sections. A summary of the treatment process is presented on Pocket Card B.3 in Appendix B.

Target Symptoms

The clinician must know what problems other than just "agitation" or "psychosis" he or she is treating. The exact description of the problematic behaviors that is gained during the assessment allows treatment to be directed toward the source of the problem. For example, an individual's agitation may consist of repetitive screaming, hitting, and resistance to bathing, and each of these three target behaviors may require a different approach. Each behavior can then be tracked individually to assess whether improvement is occurring. Sometimes, an improvement in only one or two of the multiple target behaviors is sufficient to decrease the overall level of acuity. For example, treatment of a man who is screaming and hitting because he is paranoid may produce a response of less screaming and hitting but persistent paranoia. However, the overall reduction in his agitation may be a sufficient goal.

Reversible Causes

The importance of identifying the reversible causes of agitation and psychosis is covered in Chapter 12. During treatment or palliation of the reversible causes, the use of behavioral and pharmacologic treatment strategies may still be indicated while waiting for the source of the behaviors to remit.

CLINICAL VIGNETTE

Mr. Madison, an 87-year-old man with severe Alzheimer disease, suddenly began to demonstrate combativeness during care and frequent episodes of screaming. A urinalysis indicated underlying infection, and antibiotic treatment was started. However, on the first day of treatment, he tried to attack a nurse while he was being dressed, which caused him to fall out of his wheelchair so that he sustained a contusion to his arm. He was subsequently started on a low dose of an antipsychotic to calm him. After his course of antibiotics, the antipsychotic was discontinued, without any further behavioral problems.

Environment

An environmental or behavioral plan is a nonpharmacologic way of reducing the frequency and intensity of disruptive behaviors. Some plans work by identifying and responding to the needs of the patient that require attention, such as relieving hunger, thirst, or discomfort from soiled clothing or excessive heat, cold, or noise. Individuals with dementia often have a reduced stress threshold, so even minor upsets or unmet needs can trigger an excessive reaction. Other plans use stimuli or reinforcements to shape behavior in a desired direction. Several examples of these approaches are illustrated in the following clinical vignettes.

CLINICAL VIGNETTE

Problem: Resistance to Care and Abusive Language
Mr. Green resisted attempts by the staff to dress him in the

morning. He would become combative and verbally abusive when the aides attempted to get him ready for breakfast. Otherwise, he was relatively calm during the rest of the day. The staff identified early morning as a particularly difficult time for him, and the decision was made to postpone attempts to dress him until after breakfast. This change reduced the morning struggle. The staff ignored his abusive language and praised him when he spoke more reasonably. Mr. Green's family members later told the staff that, before developing dementia, Mr. Green always enjoyed spending several hours in the morning drinking coffee and reading the paper before getting ready for work. The staff started to provide Mr. Green with a cup of decaffeinated coffee and a paper with breakfast. His resistance to care improved markedly because the behavioral approach was replicating what was once a very familiar and relaxing routine for Mr. Green.

CLINICAL VIGNETTE

Problem: Intrusive Wandering, Agitation, and Physical Aggression

Ms. Allen was constantly going into the nursing station and attempting to take things from the front desk. She would ask questions repeatedly despite being provided with answers. When the staff shooed her away, she became furious and would begin cursing the staff and damaging items. The staff members then learned that Ms. Allen used to be an executive secretary at a prestigious corporation, and they wondered whether her behaviors were an attempt to "work." To accommodate Ms. Allen, they designated a corner of the desk at the nursing station as Ms. Allen's workspace and stocked it with extra papers, tape dispensers, envelopes, and magazines. Whenever Ms. Allen approached the desk, she would be "asked" by staff to help with some work by sitting in her "desk." This request mollified Ms. Allen, who seemed to enjoy moving papers around and making suggestions to the unit secretary. She also enjoyed the verbal banter with the nurses and the other staff members who frequently stopped by the desk.

In each of these vignettes, the behavioral plan took into account that patients' previous lifestyles and personality characteristics, and it attempted to provide a more accommo-dating schedule or environment to decrease triggers, to increase structure, and to redirect behaviors into a more stim-ulating and productive direction. Behavioral plans require a great deal of creativity, flexibility, and patience on the part of staff. Several examples of environmental and behavioral strategies are listed in Table 13.1. Sometimes, however, the

TABLE 13.1. Environmental and Behavioral Strategies for Common Target Behaviors

Target behavior	Strategies
Agitation during caregiving	Use a calm, nonthreatening manner
	Select an optimal time
	Provide soothing or relaxing stimulation beforehand
Repetitive screaming, requests, or complaints	Identify unmet needs (e.g., pain, need for toileting)
	Provide increased socialization
	Reduce overstimulation in environment
Intrusive wandering	Provide safe and stimulating areas to wander
	Distract with meaningful activities and socialization
	Enhance personal space with familiar photographs or other items
Verbal abuse	Redirect to other topics and activities
	Reinforce nonabusive language with praise
	Provide meaningful activities and socialization
Inappropriate touching	Set limits and redirect to other activities
	Provide adequate, appropriate physical stimulation
Paranoid ideation	Interact in nonthreatening manner
	Avoid challenging beliefs but empathize with fear
	Redirect onto less threatening topics
Repetitive somatic complaints	Identify unmet needs (adequate pain control?)
	Provide positive sensory stimulation
	Give one-to-one contact to reassure and reduce anxiety

environment is simply not safe or structured enough for a particular person, and a move must be considered.

Individual psychotherapy as part of the behavioral plan can be helpful, depending on the degree of dementia. The short-term memory impairment may limit an individual's ability to acquire insight and cognitive skills and to carry them into future sessions. A more practical approach involves supportive psychotherapy in the here and now to provide socialization, anxiety reduction, and rudimentary problem solving. Neuropsychologic testing helps determine the feasibility and best approach to individual psychotherapy.

 TIP

Although the use of behavioral techniques can seem quite involved, always begin by using your common sense. Think about the patient and the situation, and ask yourself several of the following basic questions: What does the patient need? What is bothering him or her? What might make him or her feel better? The best environmental and behavioral plans are often based on the practical, intuitive, and empathic ways in which nurses and aides can comfort and care for troubled patients.

PSYCHOPHARMACOLOGIC APPROACHES TO TREAT AGITATION AND PSYCHOSIS

The use of psychopharmacology to treat agitation and psychosis ideally occurs after a thorough assessment has been completed, any reversible problems have been addressed, and environmental and behavioral strategies have been implemented. The selection of an appropriate pharmacologic agent is guided by several factors as follows:

- What are the target symptoms?
- Is a comorbid psychiatric disorder that is underlying the symptoms present?
- Has any particular agent worked well or not worked in the past?
- Is the patient taking other medications that pose risks for drug interactions?
- What side effects should be avoided?

Of particular importance is the presence of a psychiatric disorder or symptom cluster that underlies the agitation or psychosis. For example, psychotic symptoms always necessitate the use of an antipsychotic agent, whereas depressive features that are associated with agitation or psychosis suggest the use of an antidepressant. Not every case will fit neatly into one of these categories, but they provide a means for approaching a clinical presentation initially and then a method for reevaluating it when the symptoms persist.

Nearly every type of psychopharmacologic agent has been used to treat agitation, whereas only antipsychotic agents are used to treat psychosis. A clinical presentation that involves both agitation and psychosis requires, at the very least, the use of an antipsychotic. When the clinician is selecting a first-line agent, he or she should always determine whether anything the individual has taken in the past has worked well, has failed to work, or has caused side effects. The clinician should also anticipate the likely side effects for each potential agent and should consider their impact on the patient. For example, a more stimulating medication may not be desirable in a hyperactive patient, whereas a more sedating agent may be hazardous for a patient with an unsteady gait and a high risk of falls. Medications that strongly induce or inhibit key hepatic isoenzymes can disrupt the effectiveness of, or can cause toxicity with, medications such as warfarin, anticonvulsants, and tricyclic antidepressants. In patients with brittle diabetes, medications that cause a risk of glucose intolerance should be used only with extra caution and close monitoring; in patients with severe cardiac disease, medications that can significantly elevate the heart rate, alter blood pressure, slow down cardiac conduction, or elevate triglyceride levels should not be prescribed.

The spectrum of potential psychopharmacologic agents is broad, including the following:

Anxiolytics;
Antidepressants;
Beta-blockers;
Acetylcholinesterase (AChE) inhibitors;
Mood stabilizers;
Antipsychotics.

Although each category is reviewed here, the reader should realize by the end of the chapter that the most broad-spectrum and efficacious choices are the atypical antipsychotics. Table 13.2 contains a list of the main psychopharmacologic medications and dosing strategies used to treat agitation and psychosis (dosing for AChE inhibitors is presented in Chap-

TABLE 13.2. Recommended Psychopharmacologic Agents for Agitation and Psychosis Associated with Dementia

Name	Starting Dose	Dose Range (mg/d)
Antipsychotics (atypical)		
Clozapine (Clozaril)	6.25–12 mg	25–350
Risperidone (Risperdal)	0.25–0.5 mg	0.25–2.0
Olanzapine (Zyprexa)	2.5–5 mg	2.5–10
Quetiapine (Seroquel)	25–50 mg	25–400
Antipsychotics (conventional)		
Haloperidol (Haldol)	0.25–0.5 mg	0.5–2
Mood stabilizers		
Divalproex (Depakote, Depakene)	125 mg b.i.d.–t.i.d.	500–1500
Carbamazepine (Tegretol)	50–100 mg b.i.d.	100–500
Gabapentin (Neurontin)	50–100 mg q.d.–b.i.d.	200–1200
Anxiolytics		
Lorazepam (Ativan)	0.25–0.5 mg	0.25–2
Oxazepam (Serax)	7.5–10 mg	15–45
Alprazolam (Xanax)	0.125–0.25 mg	0.25–1
Buspirone (BuSpar)	5 mg b.i.d.	10–60

Abbreviations: b.i.d., twice daily; q.d., every day; t.i.d., three times a day.

ter 7 and antidepressants in Chapter 14). The reader should keep in mind that this table provides guidelines for dosing based on common practice, but higher or lower doses may be used clinically, depending on the situation.

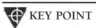 KEY POINT

The goal of medication management for agitation or psychosis is to achieve symptom remission at a given dose of an agent that is tolerated by the patient. After the initial doses are given, an improvement in agitation ideally should occur within hours to days, depending on the agent. Antipsychotic effects can take several weeks, however. After symptomatic improvement begins, further titration may be needed to maximize this benefit without causing side effects, or the dose may need to be adjusted because of side effects. This process can take several weeks.

Anxiolytics

The anxiolytics include the *benzodiazepines* and *buspirone* (BuSpar). The *benzodiazepines* are believed to work by enhancing the effects of the inhibitory neurotransmitter γ-aminobutyric acid. They have several advantages in treating individuals with dementia and agitation, including the fact that they work quickly (within minutes to hours) and safely and that they are easy to dose and dispense. Benzodiazepines are best for (a) treating episodic agitation, anxiety, or panic; (b) initial but short-term treatment (1 to 4 weeks) of agitation, anxiety or panic symptoms, mania, and insomnia; and (c) behavioral emergencies. For long-term control of agitation, however, the clinician should switch patients to other psychopharmacologic agents, particularly mood stabilizers or antipsychotics. The reason for this lies in their potential for accumulating side effects to which frail, elderly patients with dementia are especially vulnerable, such as oversedation, ataxia, falls, anterograde amnesia, confusion, and decreased function. These side effects are of particular concern with the use of the long-acting benzodiazepines, such as clonazepam (Klonopin) or diazepam (Valium). Conversely, short-acting agents, such as triazolam (Halcion) and alprazolam (Xanax), have been associated with paradoxical agitation and rebound symptoms.

The most commonly used benzodiazepines include lorazepam (Ativan), alprazolam, diazepam, oxazepam (Serax), chlordiazepoxide (Librium), and clonazepam. Some common sleeping pills are triazolam (Halcion), flurazepam (Dalmane), and temazepam (Restoril). Because of its simpler metabolism, its short (but not too short) half-life, and its familiarity among physicians and nurses, lorazepam generally is the most widely prescribed agent in long-term care facilities and hospital and emergency department settings.

Buspirone, a novel antianxiety medication that works as a partial serotonin agonist, has an onset of action that is similar to that of antidepressants, requiring 10 days to 2 weeks or longer for improvement to occur. Therefore, it cannot be used like benzodiazepines on an as-needed basis. It has mainly been used to treat generalized anxiety disorder, but it can also augment other antidepressants in the treatment of depression and obsessive-compulsive disorder. In general, it is well tolerated, and its common side effects include nausea, vomiting, headache, and dizziness. When it is used to treat agitation, the dosing is begun at 5 mg twice daily and is increased by 5-mg to 10-mg increments to a range of 30 to 60 mg per day in two or three divided doses. The most common dose range in dementia tends to be 20 to 30 mg per day (10 mg two or three times daily or 15 mg twice daily). Buspirone is best when used in patients with mild to moderate agitation who have a clear anxiety component underlying their symptoms. Because the results generally are modest, many clinicians use buspirone in combination with other medications, particularly the selective serotonin reuptake inhibitor (SSRI) antidepressants.

Antidepressant Medications

Antidepressants are commonly used to treat depression associated with dementia and agitation with depressive features (e.g., irritability, negativity, weepiness, impaired sleep and appetite). The mechanism of action of the SSRI antidepressants used to treat behavioral problems that are independent of depression may be related to their ability to reverse deficient serotonergic activity, which has been associated with aggression, psychosis, and sleep disturbances. Similar efficacy for antidepressants that enhance noradrenergic and dopaminergic functioning has not been established. With any antidepressant, the risk of actually triggering agitation and psychosis because of excess stimulation must be considered, especially when dopaminergic activity is increased. Because of its sedating properties, trazodone (Desyrel) is the most widely studied antidepressant treatment for agitation. Trazodone may be started at a dose of 25 to 50 mg daily and then increased to 100 to 300 mg daily in two to three divided doses. The most common side effect of trazodone is sedation, a property that is exploited in the treatment of agitation. Less common side effects are dizziness; headache; orthostasis; cardiac irritability (at higher doses); and, rarely, priapism.

Beta-Blockers

Beta-blockers are sometimes used to reduce agitation and aggression in patients with dementia and brain injury. The rationale for their use is based on the belief that aggression is associated with a heightened reactivity to noradrenergic stimulation. Their use as single or adjunctive agents was more common before the advent of the atypical antipsychotic medications, but they have now become third-line or fourth-line choices. Beta-blockers can also be used to treat akathisia (motor restlessness) that occurs as a side effect of antipsychotics. Severe akathisia can, if left untreated, cause agitation. Side effects of beta-blockers occur infrequently, and they are dose related. The most common are hypotension, bradycardia, depression, lethargy, bronchospasm, glucose dysregulation, disorientation, and sexual dysfunction. Given these side effects, beta-blockers should be used with particular caution in individuals with diabetes, asthma, chronic obstructive pulmonary disease, and congestive heart failure.

Acetylcholinesterase Inhibitors

Behavioral problems in Alzheimer disease and other dementias may be related to cholinergic deficits. Studies with donepezil, rivastigmine, and galantamine have indicated that individuals on these AChE inhibitors demonstrate fewer behavioral problems over time compared with individuals on a placebo. Despite this association, more research is needed to determine whether the AChE inhibitors actually treat agitation or merely reduce its prevalence. Lacking these data, AChE inhibitors should not be used as first-line agents; rather, they should be administered with other psychopharmacologic agents as adjunctive therapy (see Chapter 7).

Mood Stabilizers

Mood stabilizers have been used to treat bipolar disorder, recurrent depression, impulse control disorder, and aggression associated with brain impairment. Lithium was the first mood stabilizer, and it has been a staple of psychiatric care for more than three decades. Anticonvulsants, in addition to being used to treat seizure and movement disorders, neuropathic pain, and migraine headaches, have been used as mood stabilizers for the past 15 years. For individuals with dementia, mood stabilizers may be useful for treating agitation that involves manic features or underlying bipolar disorder, severe impulsivity, aggression, and disinhibition. The mood stabilizers do not treat the psychotic symptoms directly, but they may reduce the associated agitation.

Because of its side effects and narrow therapeutic window, *lithium carbonate* (Eskalith, Lithobid) is often not used in agitated elderly individuals with dementia. When it is used, the dosing is begun at 150 mg once or twice daily and is then titrated to clinical effect, which usually occurs in the range of

300 to 1,200 mg daily. Checking blood levels routinely is imperative, especially after dose changes or the addition of medications known to affect lithium levels.

Blood levels should be kept between 0.6 and 1.0 mEq per L, although some individuals may respond at lower levels. Higher levels, although they can bring an individual perilously close to toxicity, are sometimes required to treat bipolar disorder. The common side effects of lithium carbonate include sedation, tremor, and diarrhea. The gastrointestinal side effects can sometimes be managed by switching from regular lithium carbonate to a slow-release or controlled-release preparation or to liquid lithium citrate. Renal and thyroid tests should be checked before the medication is begun to establish a baseline and then every 4 to 6 months thereafter because of the risk of damage to both organs. Many medications, especially nonsteroidal antiinflammatory drugs, can affect lithium levels, generally by increasing them.

Valproic acid, which is dispensed as *divalproex sodium* (Depakote, Depakene), has demonstrated both clinical efficacy for treating the agitation associated with dementia and a relatively safe profile in both case series and placebo-controlled trials. It has also been shown to be effective in augmenting other psychopharmacologic agents, particularly the antipsychotics. Divalproex comes in a variety of preparations, including enterically coated and extended-release tablets, sprinkles, and syrup. The dosing is begun at 125 mg orally twice daily and is increased in 125-mg increments to a usual range of 375 to 1,500 mg daily in two or three doses. Three to 4 days after each dose increase, blood levels should be drawn before the morning dose and checked; the aim should be for levels in the range of 40 to 90 μg per mL. Divalproex levels should be checked every 4 months once an individual is stable. The most common side effects include gastrointestinal intolerance, sedation, and ataxia. Hepatotoxicity, thrombocytopenia, and pancreatitis are less common, but critical, side effects. For this reason, the clinician should be sure to obtain baseline liver function tests, an amylase level, and a complete blood count and then to monitor these levels every 4 to 6 months while the patient continues on treatment with valproic acid.

Carbamazepine (Tegretol), like divalproex, has demonstrated efficacy for treating agitation in both case series and placebo-controlled trials. The dosing starts at 50 to 100 mg daily, with typical dose ranges of 100 to 500 mg per day. The dose should be titrated to clinical effect, not to blood level, although safe levels for elderly individuals with dementia are in the range of 3 to 8 μg per mL. Some common side effects are sedation, ataxia, gastrointestinal intolerance, and tremor; less common, but critical, side effects include the syndrome of inappropriate secretion of antidiuretic hormone (SIADH), hepatotoxicity, bone marrow suppression, and Stevens–Johnson syndrome. In addition to checking carbamazepine levels every 1 to 2 weeks during the first 6 to 8 weeks of treatment and every 4 months once the patient is stable, liver function tests and a complete blood count should be checked at baseline and then every 6 months thereafter. Carbamazepine can strongly induce its own hepatic metabolism and those of numerous other medications, thereby creating an increased risk of drug toxicity. For example, carbamazepine plasma levels can be decreased by other anticonvulsants and theophylline and increased by oral antifungal medications, macrolide antibiotics, calcium channel blockers, fluoxetine, and cimetidine. Carbamazepine may also induce the metabolism of warfarin and other anticonvulsants, leading to decreased plasma levels of these. Extra monitoring of blood levels is required with all of these combinations.

Other anticonvulsants, such as *gabapentin* (Neurontin), *lamotrigine* (Lamictal), and *topiramate* (Topamax), have demonstrated a limited efficacy in treating agitation. Gabapentin is generally as well tolerated as divalproex, and the side effects, including sedation and ataxia, are similar. One small clinical trial found that gabapentin in a dose range of 200 to 1,200 mg daily was moderately efficacious in treating behavioral disorders. The main concern with the use of lamotrigine is the possibility of severe, life-threatening skin rashes. Topiramate appears to be well tolerated in younger individuals, with the bonus that it does not promote weight gain, but almost no data have been published on its use in individuals with dementia.

Antipsychotic Medications

Antipsychotic medications are the best studied and most widely used medications for treating both agitation and psychosis. Researchers have long known that excessive dopaminergic activity is associated with agitation, and all antipsychotics are believed to work by blocking dopamine receptors. Until the late 1980s, the medications that are now called the *conventional* antipsychotics were the only choices for treatment of psychotic disorders and agitation and psychosis in individuals with dementia. The most popular conventional agents included chlorpromazine (Thorazine), thioridazine (Mellaril), and haloperidol (Haldol). Despite their widespread use, efficacy studies for agitation and psychosis in dementia using conventional antipsychotics were not impressive, revealing a general improvement rate only 18% greater than that seen with a placebo. Even when conventional antipsychotics are dosed appropriately, their use poses considerable risks in older, frail individuals due to the frequent occurrence of extrapyramidal symptoms (EPS) and anticholinergic side effects and the increased risk of tardive dyskinesia (TD) with age and exposure (see Chapter 4 for clinical definitions of EPS and TD). Rates of EPS may approach 70% in older individuals, and the risk of TD in the first year of exposure is nearly 40%. Despite these factors, the conventional antipsychotics are still widely used, partly because of their familiarity to many clinicians.

Atypical antipsychotics were first introduced in the late 1980s with *clozapine* (Clozaril), and six are currently approved by the United States Food and Drug Administration for use in the United States. These antipsychotics were labeled "atypical" because of several distinct differences and advantages over previous agents as follows: (a) they block dopamine receptors and a subset of serotonin receptors; (b) they produce significantly lower rates of EPS and negligible rates of TD; and (c) they demonstrate overall improved efficacy in treating psychosis, especially with respect to the negative symptoms in schizophrenia (e.g., emotional and social withdrawal, blunted affect, impoverished speech). Although these agents are only approved for schizophrenia, they have been studied in, and are used widely, for the treatment of agitation and psychosis in dementia and bipolar disorder. They produce variable side effects, but, in general, patients taking these must be monitored for sedation, dizziness, impaired gait and risk of falls, EPS, weight gain, headache, elevated triglyceride levels, glucose dysfunction and increased risk of diabetes, and even paradoxical agitation. For all of these agents, checking a baseline fasting glucose level and then periodically following it during treatment are prudent. EPS remains the side effect of greatest concern in the elderly, although, at therapeutic doses, the rate of EPS in all atypical antipsychotics is not significantly greater than that seen with the use of a placebo. The dosing range for older patients with schizophrenia tends to be higher than that for dementia, whereas the range for patients with Parkinson disease tends to be lower. In many cases, the atypical agents are used in combination with other psychopharmacologic agents, including divalproex sodium, lorazepam, antidepressants, and AChE inhibitors.

As was noted, *clozapine* was the first atypical agent on the market. Despite its good efficacy, it can produce strong sedative effects, weight gain, anticholinergic effects, glucose dysregulation, and diabetes, and it has a risk of agranulocytosis as well. These side effects, as well as the need to perform a complete blood count every 1 to 2 weeks, limit its use in older individuals with dementia. The use of *risperidone* (Risperdal), with a target dose range of 0.5 to 1.5 mg per day in a single dose or divided doses, has been extensively studied for the treatment of agitation and psychosis associated with dementia. Risperidone generally is the least sedating of the atypical agents commonly used for patients with dementia, and it is not strongly associated with glucose intolerance or a risk of diabetes. Dose-related increases in prolactin levels may occur, although without a clear association with specific side effects. *Olanzapine* (Zyprexa), the third atypical antipsychotic to come on the market, is also used to treat agitation and psychosis in dementia, with a target dose range of 5 to 10 mg in a single bedtime dose or divided doses. In clinical trials, olanzapine was not associated with EPS. The risks of sedation, weight gain, and diabetes are increased compared with other atypical agents, with the exception of clozapine. *Quetiapine* (Seroquel) is typically used in dose ranges of 50 to 200 mg daily in a single bedtime dose or in divided doses, although doses as high as 400 mg are sometimes required. Sedation and dizziness were the most common side effects in clinical trials. The risk of glucose intolerance and diabetes is minimal. Published clinical studies have not yet established dosing ranges for both *ziprasidone* (Geodon) and *aripiprazole* (Abilify) in the treatment of patients with dementia. Clinicians have been reluctant to use ziprasidone in older patients because of the increased risk of cardiac conduction delay, despite the fact that otherwise the medication has a favorable side effect profile and the lowest risk of weight gain. Aripiprazole is a novel atypical antipsychotic agent that has been called a dopamine-serotonin system stabilizer because it appears to act as a functional dopamine or serotonin *antagonist* when levels of these neurotransmitters are too high and a functional *agonist* when they are too low.

KEY POINT

After a patient has improved on a given medication, the dose should usually be maintained for 4 to 6 months before a taper is considered. If appropriate, taper slowly and watch for symptom recurrence, which may then indicate the need for long-term therapy.

Omnibus Budget Reconciliation Act Guidelines

For nursing home patients, the use of psychopharmacologic agents must adhere to the guidelines laid down by the nursing home reform amendments enacted in the Omnibus Budget Reconciliation Act (OBRA) of 1987. These reforms resulted from several years of growing concern that excessive doses of many psychiatric medications were being used in long-term care settings without clear justification, documentation, and sufficient psychiatric supervision. The OBRA guidelines for psychotropic medications are summarized on Pocket Card B.4 in Appendix B, and the dosing guidelines are listed on Pocket Card B.5. To maintain OBRA compliance, the clinician must be extremely diligent in documenting his or her clinical rationale for using a psychotropic medication, especially if the prescription is for a higher than usual dose, for an extended period of time without a taper, or for a unique indication. Adherence to OBRA guidelines is extremely important for maintaining the accreditation of a long-term care facility.

ADDRESSING THE BEHAVIORAL CRISIS

A behavioral crisis involves an individual who is engaging in physically assaultive, suicidal, or extremely unsafe behaviors that represent an immediate threat to the safety of the patient or others. Such behaviors are especially dangerous when the individual is living at home with minimal supervision or when the surrounding home environment or neighborhood is not safe. When these situations occur, the clinician may not always be near the patient, and he or she may be called at inopportune times. When the clinician does arrive on the scene, it may seem chaotic or out of control, and tensions among the family or staff may be running high. The clinician must remember to step back and assess the situation calmly. Acutely agitated patients with dementia are often reacting to feelings of fear or neglect, so the clinician should try to help them feel safe and cared for. He or she should avoid responding to the crisis in an overly reactive manner that can result in patients being overmedicated or inappropriately hospitalized or feeling that they have been punished. Irritable, dismissive, and passive-aggressive behaviors on the part of the clinician are unprofessional, unethical, and impractical since they usually make the situation worse. When the clinician feels and appears calm, professional, and self-confident, the patients then internalize some of the calmness, and the caregivers and staff try to emulate it.

The approach to behavioral emergencies represents an accelerated, more intense version of the normal assessment and treatment of agitation and psychosis. Behavioral emergencies can be addressed using to the mnemonic CALM as follows:

Calm the individual;
Assess the environment;
Limit access to unsafe places or situations;
Medicate as necessary.

Immediate intervention is required in behavioral emergencies, and it should initially be aimed at calming the individual and eliminating the situation that is producing the crisis. If the clinician is on the scene, he or she should approach the individual with a concerned expression and a friendly demeanor, speaking calmly with a soothing but firm tone. He or she should then try to distract the individual and redirect him or her into a safer area and situation or instruct a caregiver or staff member to do so. In the appropriate situations, food or drink should be offered or the individual's other needs should be addressed. Noxious triggers in the environment, such as loud or annoying voices or noises, uncomfortable physical stimuli (e.g., soiled clothes or bedding, insufficient or excessive lighting or heat), unpleasant odors, other agitated individuals, or even angry or stressed caregivers who need a break, should be identified and eliminated. Then, the clinician should make sure that the individual cannot return to the unsafe situation. This may involve removing sharp objects or potential weapons when suicidal or homicidal threats have been made and limiting access to doors or windows when escape is a risk. In a home environment, the intervention can be more challenging because the caregivers may lack assistance or they may live in unsafe neighborhoods, areas of high traffic, or near bodies of water that can be hazardous if the patient wanders away. Chapter 15 has more information on inspecting and safety-proofing a home for a patient with dementia. In life-threatening situations, emergency personnel should be called for assistance in transporting the individual to an emergency department or a psychiatric facility.

When behavioral approaches do not quickly resolve the crisis, psychopharmacologic agents can be used to calm the individual quickly and safely. Clinicians often try chemical restraints, many of which are inappropriate for older, frail individuals with dementia. Instead, most geriatric clinicians keep their approach simple, basing it on the regimen outlined in Table 13.3, which lists very few medications. Lorazepam may be the best choice in terms of fast-acting benzodiazepines because it has a simpler metabolism and a reasonable duration of action and it is a familiar and accessible medication in most settings. Both short-acting and long-acting benzodiazepines can be associated with unwanted side effects. For example, diazepam has an extremely quick onset of action, but it stays in the body for a long time, increasing the risk of side effect accumulation. Alprazolam also works quickly and relatively well, but it has been associated with paradoxical agitation and it has a short half-life that can lead to rebound symptoms within hours as the blood levels drop. Despite these admonitions, selecting a benzodiazepine that the patient is already taking or has responded to in the past is always best.

In terms of antipsychotic medications, the atypical agents are preferred, except for when intramuscular preparations are needed. In that situation, most clinicians use haloperidol because the only atypical agent with an intramuscular form is ziprasidone, which has the potential for cardiac side effects. If intramuscular haloperidol or another conventional antipsychotic is used, the patient should be switched to an atypical agent when an oral dose can be given. Patients who spit out pills can be given a liquid preparation of risperidone or an orally dissolving tablet of olanzapine or risperidone.

TABLE 13.3. Medications for Behavioral Emergencies

Strategy	Dose (range)	Comments
Benzodiazepine		
Lorazepam (Ativan)	0.5 mg p.o. or i.m. (0.25–1 mg)	Repeat as necessary after 30–60 min; p.r.n. dosing can be used every 4–12 hr
Antipsychotic		
Risperidone (Risperdal)	0.5-mg tablet, elixir, or orally-dissolving M-tab (0.25–1 mg)	Repeat doses as necessary after 30–60 min
OR		
Olanzapine (Zyprexa)	5-mg tablet or orally dissolving Zydis (2.5–5 mg)	Repeat doses as necessary after 30–60 min
OR		
Quetiapine (Seroquel)	50 mg (25–100 mg)	Repeat doses as necessary after 30–60 min
OR		
Haloperidol (Haldol)	0.5 mg i.m. (0.25–1 mg)	Start an oral atypical agent when the patient is calm.

Combine a benzodiazepine with an antipsychotic agent for severe or resistant agitation.

Alternative agent		
Trazodone (Desyrel)	50 mg (25–100 mg)	Repeat as necessary after 30–60 min

[a]**Caution:** Avoid use of triazolam (Halcion), antihistamines (diphenhydramine, hydroxyzine), chloral hydrate, chlorpromazine (Thorazine), thioridazine (Mellaril), or narcotic analgesics due to risk of oversedation, dizziness, ataxia, falls, and confusion.
Abbreviations: i.m., intramuscularly; p.o., orally; p.r.n., as needed.

CLINICAL VIGNETTE

Mrs. Ho, an 86-year-old woman with Alzheimer disease, lived with her daughter. The daughter paged her mother's psychiatrist one evening. When the psychiatrist returned her call, she was in tears. She reported that her mother attacked her with a cane and then smashed the window in the front door, trying to leave the house. Mrs. Ho was paranoid and agitated, accusing her daughter of trying to keep her in a jail.

Plan: The psychiatrist instructed the daughter over the phone to ask her mother calmly to sit down and to offer the mother her favorite snack or drink. She then tried to give her mother an extra 0.5-mg dose of risperidone. Mrs. Ho calmed down over the next hour, sat quietly in front of the television, and then fell asleep for the night. In the follow-up phone call, the psychiatrist advised the daughter to increase Mrs. Ho's daily risperidone dose to 0.5 mg twice daily.

CLINICAL VIGNETTE

Mr. Fess, a 78-year-old man with vascular dementia, insulin-dependent diabetes, and peripheral vascular disease, was admitted to a rehabilitation facility after the amputation of his left lower leg. The psychiatrist was called emergently to his unit, where he found Mr. Fess sitting on the floor naked, with feces and urine smeared around him. He was yelling and striking out at the surrounding staff and was attempting to rip a large dressing off his leg stump.

Plan: The psychiatrist observed five nurses with anxious and angry facial expressions surrounding Mr. Fess and calling out to him to calm down. They were ready to inject him with a sedative. The psychiatrist asked that the area be cleared except for two staff members, who were then asked to approach Mr. Fess calmly and quietly and to ask to help. After several minutes, Mr. Fess calmed down and began weeping. The staff then gently maneuvered him onto a towel, cleaned him up, and put a gown over him; they then cleaned the surrounding floor and cleaned and recovered his wound. No chemical restraint or psychiatric hospitalization was needed; instead, the psychiatrist simply prescribed a medication increase over the next 24 hours.

SEXUAL AGGRESSION

Sexually aggressive or inappropriate behaviors include obscene sexual comments or requests; public nudity or masturbation; and aggressive fondling, groping, or forced sexual activity. They are present in approximately 5% of individuals with dementia, although the rates on dementia units may be as high as 25%. Such behaviors in dementia are often associated with frontal and temporal lobe impairment, mania, psychosis, stroke, and head trauma. Although these behaviors create a disproportionate amount of concern and anxiety among caregivers, they can be approached and treated in the same manner as other agitated behaviors. The assessment tries to determine whether the behavior is due to excess libido, disinhibited sexual impulses, unmet sexual needs, or confusion. For example, a man with dementia who is reported to have groped a staff member may simply have been reaching out or grabbing for attention from the level of a wheelchair, thus hitting the staff member in the waist or chest area, or he may have actually been trying to satisfy a sexual urge.

The treatment of these behaviors should begin with behavioral techniques that set limits and redirect the individual into more appropriate behaviors. Eliminating the inadvertent reinforcement of these behaviors (e.g., staff members laugh at obscene comments) is also important. In some situations, the individual may be expressing unmet needs for physical stimulation or intimacy that can be gratified by partners. For example, an individual with dementia who attempts to fondle other residents could be provided with increased physical stimulation through hugs and massages during visits with his or her spouse. Problematic behaviors that appear associated with excess or disinhibited libido may respond to antidepressants that have sexual side effects, such as the SSRIs. Rarely, clinicians use estrogen or an antiandrogen steroid hormone, such as medroxyprogesterone (Provera), to reduce sexual urges. Aggressive, disinhibited, hyperactive, or hypersexual behaviors often respond well to the atypical antipsychotics and mood stabilizers.

WHEN TREATMENT FAILS

At times, behavioral disturbances or psychotic symptoms may persist or even worsen despite everyone's best efforts; such situations are frustrating for any caregiver or clinician.

CLINICAL VIGNETTE

Mr. Spitz, a 78-year-old man with Wernicke–Korsakoff encephalopathy, was a pleasant but confused individual who, most of the time, spent his days wandering up and down the hallway of the special care unit. However, one or two times a month, he would suddenly and unpredictably strike out at another resident or staff member. On one occasion, he pushed over a female resident who was using a walker, nearly causing a hip fracture. Another time, he slapped an aide in the face and attempted to push her to the ground. He had no memory of these episodes afterward and denied that he would ever do such a thing. Multiple trials of psychotropics, including benzodiazepines, mood stabilizers, antipsychotics, and combinations, resulted in sedation, but they did not extinguish these episodic behaviors.

CLINICAL VIGNETTE

Ms. Shrek, a 102-year-old nursing home resident with Alzheimer disease, spent her days sitting in a wheelchair in front of the nursing station, calling out her son Johnny's name repeatedly. Other times, she would repeat "Johnny, I need help" or "oh, oh, oh" for hours. She would stop briefly when she was asked a question but she would then start again. Her cognitive impairment was so severe that she had no insight into her behaviors, and nothing seemed to stop them. Staff members were conflicted over whether her vocalizations warranted treatment with medications, but they felt pressured to respond to the multiple complaints from other residents, families, and staff about how disruptive the verbalizations were. Trials of lorazepam, an SSRI antidepressant, and an antipsychotic medication were ineffective.

These cases illustrate some of the barriers involved in treatment-resistant symptoms. Sometimes, the symptoms are episodic but severe, and their unpredictability limits an environmental or behavioral plan. Other behaviors, such as repetitive verbalizations or vocalizations, intrusive wandering, and refusal to take medications or to cooperate with therapy or institutional rules, may not cause harm to the patient or others, but they can be extremely annoying to the other residents, caregivers, or staff. In such cases, staff members are often unsure about whether the use of psychotropic medications is justified. Other circumstances require the use of lengthy legal proceedings and family cooperation and resources to obtain a guardianship and mandated treatment plan. Behaviors that are particularly difficult to treat with medications include episodic, impulsive aggressive behaviors; repetitive disruptive vocalizations; and isolated delusions. When the clinician is facing treatment-resistant symptoms, several steps may be taken.

- Reassess for underlying medical problems, especially medication side effects or pain that may be triggering the problems.
- Reassess the diagnosis. Is an underlying depression, panic disorder, or mania that is not being treated with the appropriate medication present?
- Reassess the environment for unseen triggers.
- Reassess the environmental or behavioral plan. Perhaps elements need to be added or changed.
- Reassess the medication trials. Were adequate doses used for sufficient lengths of time? Was the patient compliant with the medication(s)? Was the caregiver dispensing it correctly? Some patients will falsely claim to be taking medications; check blood levels when possible.
- Always consider a paradoxical effect of a psychotropic medication. Is it actually exacerbating the symptoms?
- Obtain more information about the patient's underlying personality characteristics. A long-standing history of dysfunctional traits can cause persistent problems that were not fully appreciated during earlier assessments.

AUGMENTATION STRATEGIES

Several of the following pharmacologic augmentation strategies can be considered for treating agitation or psychosis when single agents are not working:

- Antipsychotic plus a benzodiazepine;
- Antipsychotic plus an antidepressant or trazodone;
- Antipsychotic plus a mood stabilizer;
- Antidepressant plus antidepressant with different receptor profile (e.g., SSRI plus mirtazapine);
- Antidepressant plus buspirone;
- Mood stabilizer plus other mood stabilizer (e.g., divalproex plus lithium);
- Mood stabilizer plus antidepressant.

Sometimes three or more agents are used. These strategies commonly include the use of AChE inhibitors. Combining two or more antipsychotics or multiple benzodiazepines should be avoided because of the increased risk of side effects. Clozapine is usually the medication of last resort. In intensive care settings, intravenous haloperidol has also been used with success. However, a dose-related risk of ventricular arrhythmias, specifically *torsade de pointes*, must be kept in mind, and it may necessitate the use of cardiac monitoring. Electroconvulsive therapy is indicated when the presence of treatment-resistant mania or psychotic depression is suspected, but it may also be considered for severe agitation that does not clearly fit into any category. When all other strategies have failed to control severe agitation, the clinician should consider moving the individual to a more structured setting, such as a dementia unit or a psychiatric hospital, for more intensive behavioral and pharmacologic management.

The clinician should remember that, even in the best medication trials, response rates are never 100%; in fact, they are rarely even 80%. Realistically, 20% to 40% of patients with agitation and/or psychosis do not respond to medication trials, even under the best of circumstances. Thus, a reassessment of the diagnosis and environment, behavioral plans, and team involvement is critical to making progress. Over time, with all of the parties working together, significant improvement can usually be achieved. Whatever the outcome, the clinician should not give up!

Assessment and Treatment of Depression and Apathy

Essential Concepts

- Depressive syndromes are seen in nearly 50% of individuals with dementia.
- Depression may have a new onset in dementia, or it may represent a recurrence of previous illness.
- Standard treatment includes psychotherapeutic techniques and antidepressant medications. Impaired sleep and appetite are frequent target symptoms.
- Apathy is a common syndrome associated with dementia; it is characterized by lack of motivation. The presence of apathy does not imply an underlying diagnosis of depression.

Depression is second only to agitation and psychosis as a significant psychiatric problem associated with dementia. It is diagnosed both as a primary illness in individuals with dementia and in association with the states of agitation and psychosis described in Chapters 12 and 13. Major depressive disorder, the most serious form of depression, is estimated to affect between 15% and 30% of all individuals with dementia. However, the total rate of all types of depressive symptoms observed in individuals with dementia is closer to 50%. These rates may be even higher in individuals with Parkinson disease and in those who have had a stroke within the previous 2 years.

Brain damage from all types of dementia creates a vulnerability to depression. In Alzheimer disease (AD), depression has been associated with neuronal loss that is greater than expected and with an increased density of plaques and tangles in the key brainstem nuclei involved in the regulation of mood, particularly the locus ceruleus, which is the center of noradrenergic function. A loss of serotonergic function in AD may further increase the risk of depression. In vascular dementia, depression is more common after damage to the left frontal regions of the brain. In addition, an association between small vessel cerebrovascular disease and depression has led to the suggested diagnosis of *vascular depression*, especially in individuals with an older age at onset. Depression has also been associated with many of the medical conditions that afflict individuals with dementia and with numerous medications, including antihypertensives, antiparkinsonian medications, beta-blockers, corticosteroids, hypoglycemic agents, narcotic analgesics, and sedative-hypnotics. Despite these associations, establishing a clear, causative link between a particular illness or medication and depression is difficult because so many other factors can be present simultaneously.

WHAT IS DEPRESSION?

When the term *depression* is used within the context of dementia, it may refer to a major depressive episode or to the atypical or less severe forms of depression often included under the label "depressive disorder, not otherwise specified." Other relevant syndromes involving depressive symptoms include dysthymic disorder, adjustment disorder, depressive personality disorder, bereavement, and bipolar disorder. To diagnose an individual with a major depressive episode according to the *Diagnostic and Statistical Manual of Mental Disorders*, Fourth Edition, Text Revision (DSM-IV-TR) criteria, an individual must have a sad or depressed mood and/or a significant decrease in interest or pleasure in almost all activities, nearly every day for most of the day, for at least 2 weeks, as well as four or more of the following features:

1. Significant change in weight or appetite;
2. Insomnia or hypersomnia nearly every day;
3. Psychomotor agitation or retardation;
4. Fatigue or loss of energy nearly every day;
5. Feelings of worthlessness or excessive or inappropriate guilt;
6. Diminished ability to think or concentrate;
7. Recurrent thoughts of death or suicidal ideation or suicidal plan or attempt.

In an attempt to account for potential diagnostic differences, DSM-IV-TR provides for the diagnosis of AD or vascular dementia with depression. Researchers have also proposed a new diagnostic entity termed *depression of AD* that includes these criteria but adds the symptoms of irritability and social isolation or withdrawal.

KEY POINT

Manic symptoms can be seen in dementia, ranging in severity from mild hyperactivity and pressured speech to gross impulsivity, disinhibition, agitation, and psychosis. These symptoms can represent either the recurrence of previous bipolar disorder or a new onset secondary to a host of medical conditions or medications. Secondary mania has been reported in association with both AD and vascular dementia, although the exact nature of this connection has yet to be elucidated.

ASSESSMENT OF DEPRESSION IN DEMENTIA

The assessment of depressive symptoms usually begins with the following key question: is this truly depression or merely dementia? Differentiating among dementia, depression, or dementia with depression can be difficult due to symptom overlap since all three entities may involve apathy, agitation, social withdrawal, impaired concentration, cognitive impairment, weight loss, and sleep disturbances. Even more complicated is the presence of depression with reversible cognitive impairment, an entity referred to as *pseudodementia*. Pseudodementia often presents like a dementia, but it must be distinguished from dementia so that the appropriate therapy can be implemented. Two basic strategies can be used to separate these diagnoses.

Step One

The first step is to reexamine the history to determine the following:

- Did current cognitive impairment exist *before* depressive symptoms? If the answer is yes, the likely diagnosis is *dementia associated with depression*.
- Are depressive symptoms present *without* clear cognitive impairment? If yes, the likely diagnosis is a *depressive disorder without dementia*.
- Did the cognitive impairment begin precipitously *after* the onset of depressive symptoms? If yes, the likely diagnosis is *pseudodementia*.

- On examination, are the alleged depressive symptoms not truly depressive? If yes, the likely diagnosis is a *dementia without depression* (consider apathy).

Depressive symptoms can also be associated with the recurrence of other psychiatric disorders, including anxiety disorders, personality disorders, and substance abuse.

Step Two

The second step is to look for clues in the mental status examination. Depressive symptoms associated with dementia often look different from the typical symptoms seen in younger individuals or in those without dementia.

Affect and Mood

Many individuals with dementia and depression do not always present with overt sadness; instead, they demonstrate uncharacteristic irritability, unreasonableness, or passivity.

 TIP

Verbal reports of affect may be inconsistent in later stages of dementia. For example, some individuals express that they feel sad at one moment, but an hour later, they do not report feeling that way. Some individuals become irritable on and off because of a temporary annoyance, but they then return to their baseline after hours or days. Although truly depressive symptoms may also fluctuate, over time, they continue to manifest with a clearly negative impact on daily function and care.

Response Style and Attitude

Individuals with dementia alone often attempt to answer questions and even to confabulate when they do not know an answer. Severely depressed individuals make poor attempts at even providing answers.

Thought Content

Depressive symptoms may include any of the following: pre-occupation with somatic symptoms or pain despite treatment with analgesics; excessive thoughts and comments about deceased relatives, personal losses, or death; and somatic delusions.

Behaviors

The presence of agitation or physical aggression should always prompt a search for underlying depression. The clinician should also look for isolative behaviors (e.g., staying in his or her room all day, refusing social contacts); noncompliance with caregiving; slow progress in rehabilitation; failure to thrive (see section titled "Poor Appetite and/or Failure to Thrive"); and indirect life-threatening behaviors, such as refusing to eat or refusing critical medications or procedures.

CLINICAL VIGNETTE

Mrs. Vines, an 82-year-old woman with moderate to severe vascular dementia and aphasia, lived in a long-term care facility. She was wheelchair bound, nearly nonverbal, and totally dependent on the staff for care. She had a feeding tube due to poor swallowing. Staff members asked for a psychiatric evaluation after they noticed that she had stopped smiling at them during bathing and that she had begun to have episodes of crying. At times, they heard her moaning in her room for no apparent reason. Mrs. Vines was unable to communicate her feelings, and her cognitive impairment prevented her from even fully understanding them. A clinical interview could yield little information because she was nonverbal. However, changes in behavior and episodes of crying suggested underlying depression. The proof came when these episodes ceased following the use of antidepressant medication.

 TIP

Individuals with sudden and frequent fits of crying may have *pseudobulbar palsy,* also called *emotional incontinence,* in which brain damage has disrupted their control of emotional expression. Such individuals may appear to be depressed, but the spontaneity and frequency of crying attacks, especially when they occur in response to being startled, or the absence of other depressive symptoms should point the clinician away from the diagnosis of depression.

Other Assessment Tools

Although the differential diagnosis for depression and dementia relies mostly on the mental status examination, several assessment tools can be useful. The most helpful neuropsychologic tests involve those for memory acquisition and retrieval. Whereas depression can reduce scores on these tests, dementia fundamentally impairs them. When dementia and depression occur together, the memory test scores may be even worse. Structural brain scans are not particularly useful for distinguishing AD from late-life depression because both may involve similar nondiagnostic findings, such as diffuse atrophy, ventricular enlargement, and leukoariosis. Positron emission tomography scans may demonstrate decreased cerebral glucose metabolism in the frontal and right hemispheres in depression, while parietal lobe hypometabolism is observed in AD.

Reports from caregivers can aid the clinician in reaching a diagnosis of depression in dementia, especially information regarding appetite, sleep, weight, and activity levels. The Geriatric Depression Scale, or GDS, is a self-report instrument that can be helpful in early stages of disease when the individual is still a relatively reliable historian (i.e., he or she is able to score at least 15 on the Mini-Mental State Examination). In the moderate to severe stages of dementia, however, the Hamilton Rating Scale for Depression, or HAM-D, and the Cornell Scale for Depression in Dementia are more practical because they are based on the clinical interview and observation and caregiver input. Some clinicians also use the 24-item Dementia Mood Assessment Scale, which incorporates both observation and a semistructured patient interview. A summary of the assessment process for depression associated with dementia, including a depression symptom checklist, is found in Appendix C on Pocket Cards C.1 and C.2. Sources for the depression scales can be found in the "Suggested Readings" section of this book.

DEPRESSION AND THE RISK OF DEMENTIA

In his 1915 textbook on psychopathology, Emil Kraepelin first suggested an association between depression and the later development of dementia. Since then, several large studies have confirmed this link, although the causal relationship is not understood. One theory suggests that, during depression, higher than normal levels of corticosteroids, or stress hormones, eventually cause brain damage. Other evidence of the depression–dementia link comes from associations found between late-onset depression and the APOE4 allele, which is a risk factor for the development of AD.

Pseudodementia refers to a syndrome of cognitive deficits that are associated with depression and that improve with treatment. The cognitive impairment is usually mild, involving problems with attention, recall, motor speed, and syntactic complexity. Compared with major depression without cognitive impairment, depression with pseudodementia tends to be more severe; it is often recurrent; and it involves more motor retardation, hopelessness, helplessness, and psychosis. Aphasia and apraxia are typically not seen. A history of depression is often present. Twenty percent to 60% of the depressed elderly develop a reversible dementia syndrome. The increased risk of developing a true dementia in individuals with pseudodementia is impressive—in one study of individuals hospitalized for depression, 43% with pseudodementia later developed irreversible dementia, compared with 12% of those who had depression alone.

 TIP

In the clinical interview, individuals with pseudodementia are often less cooperative with mental status testing and less reactive to pleasurable or interesting stimuli. In addition, their abilities may fluctuate with their level of motivation. Individuals with dementia display more consistent cognitive impairment with little fluctuation.

TREATMENT OF DEPRESSION ASSOCIATED WITH DEMENTIA

Several unique challenges are encountered when one is treating depression associated with dementia. The degree of cognitive impairment poses an immediate limitation to the efficacy of various forms of psychotherapy. Insight-oriented therapy becomes impossible if an individual cannot retain insights from one appointment to the next. Progressive aphasia makes communication with the therapist increasingly difficult. Even overlearned coping skills can be compromised by impairment in executive function. As a result, the psychologic skills that are required for talk therapy to overcome depression fade away over time. However, adapting cognitive and/or behavioral techniques to benefit individuals with mild to moderate dementia is possible. In addition, improving the problem-solving skills of their caregivers may benefit depressed individuals with dementia. Some other beneficial forms of psychotherapy are supportive individual and group therapy, structured activities, recreational therapy, and increased caregiver support.

CLINICAL VIGNETTE

Mr. Jackson, a 78-year-old man with dementia who lived in a nursing home, suffered from chronic loneliness that evolved into a depressive state that was characterized by episodes of crying, loss of appetite, and social isolation. His poor memory made remembering his weekly meetings with the social worker impossible. Knowing that he loved jazz and used to play in a small band, the staff arranged for him to meet with the music therapist. Although he could not remember the therapist between sessions, he clearly responded to the music and the opportunity to play several percussion instruments. His family also made arrangements to visit him more often. Mr. Jackson improved moderately over the course of several weeks.

Such therapeutic approaches have variable results, but they should always be incorporated into the treatment. Patients with severe dementia live in the present, and they do not retain memories or new skills from activity to activity. Instead, therapy provides comfort; support; and social, physical, and sensory stimulation to gratify their basic needs and to tap into long-time interests and personality strengths.

Antidepressant Therapy

When depressive symptoms do not respond adequately to nonpharmacologic approaches or when the symptoms are severe and potentially life threatening, antidepressant medications are needed. The same medications used in younger individuals and those without dementia are used to treat patients with dementia, with the same adage as with all elderly patients—"start low, go slow, *but go*." As with all geriatric patients, a full antidepressant response may take 6 to 8 weeks to achieve a therapeutic dose. In addition, different

TABLE 14.1. Dosing for Recommended Antidepressants in Dementia

Antidepressant	Starting dose	Range
Selective serotonin reuptake inhibitors		
Fluoxetine (Prozac)	10 mg	10–40 mg/d
Sertraline (Zoloft)	25 mg	25–100 mg/d
Paroxetine (Paxil)	10 mg	10–40 mg/d
Citalopram (Celexa)	10 mg	10–40 mg/d
Escitalopram (Lexapro)	5 mg	5–20 mg/d
Other antidepressants		
Bupropion (Wellbutrin)	50 mg b.i.d./ SR, 100 mg q.d.	100–300 mg/d
Mirtazapine (Remeron)	7.5–15 mg q.h.s.	15–45 mg/d
Venlafaxine (Effexor)	25 mg b.i.d./XR, 37.5 mg b.i.d.	75–225 mg/d
Nefazodone (Serzone)	50 mg q.h.s.	100–300 mg
Tricyclic antidepressants		
Nortriptyline (Pamelor)	10 mg q.h.s.	10–100 mg/d
Desipramine (Norpramin)	10 mg q.h.s.	10–100 mg/d
Psychostimulants		
Methylphenidate (Ritalin)	5 mg every morning	5–20 mg b.i.d. (every morning and every noon)

Abbreviations: b.i.d., twice daily; q.d., daily; q.h.s., every night; SR, sustained release; XR, extended release.

medications may bring very different results, in terms of both efficacy and side effects. For caregivers and physicians to identify these side effects early in the course of treatment is critical because they can decrease compliance and can even worsen the cognitive impairment. Each type of antidepressant is reviewed in this chapter; dosing strategies are listed in Table 14.1. Basic treatment strategies for depression associated with dementia are summarized on Pocket Card C.3 in Appendix C.

Selective Serotonin Reuptake Inhibitors

The selective serotonin reuptake inhibitors (SSRIs) are considered first-line agents for treating depression associated with dementia. As their name indicates, SSRIs work by blocking the reuptake of serotonin. They are the most widely prescribed psychiatric medications and clearly the most widely used antidepressants in all geriatric populations due to their easy dosing, excellent safety profiles, and efficacy, which is equal to that of the tricyclic antidepressants (TCAs) (once considered the gold standards) but without the same degree of side effects. The SSRIs currently on the market include fluoxetine (Prozac), fluvoxamine (Luvox), sertraline (Zoloft), paroxetine (Paxil), citalopram (Celexa), and its enantiomer escitalopram (Lexapro). No SSRI has been demonstrated to have an efficacy that is superior to that of another for treating depression associated with dementia.

SSRIs are typically dosed once daily in the morning because of their stimulating effects, although paroxetine has a greater potential for sedation so it is also dosed in the evening. As with other antidepressants, the clinical effect may be seen after 10 days to 2 weeks, but it may take as long as 6 to 8 weeks to manifest fully. The starting doses can be increased if minimal or no response is seen by 2 to 3 weeks. The common side effects include insomnia, anorexia, weight loss, diarrhea, and agitation, and some individuals experience sedation and weight gain. With its long half-life, fluoxetine and its active metabolite norfluoxetine, which has an even longer half-life, may be used in cases in which compliance is a problem. A form of fluoxetine that is taken weekly is also available; it may improve compliance in some patients. Conversely, this long half-life may become problematic when a side effect or drug–drug interaction occurs and resolution is delayed while blood levels fall slowly. Paroxetine has a short half-life with no active metabolites, and it clears the most quickly, if clearance is necessary. Sertraline, citalopram, and escitalopram may have fewer drug–drug interactions. Fluvoxamine is mainly used in older individuals to treat obsessive-compulsive disorder.

MIRTAZAPINE (REMERON)

Mirtazapine is a novel antidepressant that stimulates serotonin and norepinephrine release. It also has antagonistic properties at two serotonin receptors, $5\text{-}HT_2$ and $5\text{-}HT_3$. Therefore, it enhances serotonergic function while avoiding the common SSRI side effects of anxiety, irritability, sexual dysfunction, and nausea and/or vomiting. Because of its selective profile, mirtazapine is often used to target symptoms of insomnia, poor appetite, and weight loss associated with depression. Mirtazapine is also used to augment other antidepressants, particularly the SSRIs, and to reverse the common SSRI side effects previously mentioned. Dosing starts at 7.5 to 15 mg taken at bedtime (because of its sedating effects), with titration in 15-mg increments to a range of 15 to 45 mg per day. Mirtazapine tends to be well tolerated, with common side effects of sedation and weight gain. Mirtazapine also comes in an orally dissolving tablet (Remeron SolTab).

VENLAFAXINE (EFFEXOR)

Venlafaxine inhibits the reuptake of both serotonin and norepinephrine. Dosing starts at 18.75 to 37.5 mg twice daily for regular venlafaxine and at 37.5 mg once or twice daily for the extended release formula. The dose should be titrated to a range of 75 to 225 mg per day. Venlafaxine's common side effects include sedation, nausea, and increased blood pressure. The patient's blood pressure should be monitored daily for a week after both the initiation of treatment and each dose increase. Although the typical increase in blood pressure is usually small (5 to 10 mm Hg on average) and it may be partially mitigated by the extended release formula, it can be higher in some individuals; therefore, it should be closely tracked in individuals with underlying hypertension. Venlafaxine is a good first-line or second-line agent for SSRI nonresponders, and it is often used to augment mirtazapine and bupropion.

Bupropion (Wellbutrin)

Bupropion is believed to enhance both serotonergic and dopaminergic transmission, although the exact mechanism is not known. Given its dopaminergic properties, bupropion often has stimulating effects that are useful for treating apathy and depressive states associated with fatigue. However, this stimulating effect may also precipitate anxiety and agitation or may exacerbate preexisting problems in patients with dementia. Dosing starts at 37.5 to 50 mg twice daily for regular bupropion and at 100 mg daily for the sustained release formula. The dose can be titrated to a range of 100 to 300 mg per day, divided into two or three doses (two doses with the sustained release formula). The common side effects include agitation; insomnia; and muscle weakness, especially in the legs. A small increase in the risk of seizures is seen, especially if the patient has a preexisting seizure disorder; a history of seizures; or a potential seizure focus, such as that due to a stroke. To avoid increasing this risk, single doses should be limited to no more than 150 mg.

Nefazodone (Serzone)

Nefazodone (Serzone) is an SSRI, but it has 5-HT$_{2A}$ receptor antagonism. It can be slightly sedating, and it may target symptoms of insomnia and anxiety. Dosing starts at 50 mg twice daily, with titration in 50-mg increments to a range of 200 to 300 mg per day. The common side effects are sedation, nausea, dry mouth, and dizziness. Recently, hepatic failure has been reported as a rare but serious side effect. The related medication trazodone (Desyrel) is not widely used as an anti-depressant because therapeutic doses are associated with excess sedation.

Tricyclic Antidepressants

TCAs used to be the mainstay of antidepressant treatment. Today, however, their use has decreased dramatically in the elderly because other medication choices have equal efficacy with increased safety and better side effect profiles. The current Omnibus Budget Reconciliation Act of 1987 guidelines for long-term care discourage use of the TCAs because of their common side effect profile, including the following: orthostatic hypotension, sedation, strong anticholinergic effects, and slowed cardiac conduction. The anticholinergic side effects are particularly common with amitriptyline (Elavil), imipramine (Tofranil), doxepin (Sinequan), and clomipramine (Anafranil), making their use contraindicated in patients with dementia. TCA use in the elderly with dementia is commonly restricted to nortriptyline (Pamelor) and desipramine (Norpramin) because of their lower risk of problematic side effects compared with that of the other TCAs. Neurologists sometimes use TCAs in low doses to treat neuropathic pain and migraine headache, but, even at low doses, they can cause sedation, anticholinergic effects, and confusion.

TCAs are, therefore, reserved for individuals with dementia who have failed other antidepressants or who have a history of a particularly good response to a TCA. Before prescribing any TCA, however, reviewing a baseline electrocardiogram is critical. The presence of existing cardiac conduction delays (e.g., heart block, bundle branch block, QTc interval greater than 0.44) are usually contraindications to TCA use. For treatment with either nortriptyline or desipramine, 10 to 25 mg should be started at bedtime (given the potential for sedation) and should then be titrated to an initial dose of 25 to 50 mg. The patient should then be observed for both therapeutic effect and side effects for 2 to 3 weeks before further titration is considered. The therapeutic range for nortriptyline is 50 to 150 mg per day (therapeutic blood levels of 50 to 150 ng per mL); for desipramine, it is 50 to 200 mg per day (therapeutic blood levels of 115 to 200 ng/mL or greater than 155 ng per mL). The blood levels should be checked at steady state, approximately 5 to 7 days after a plateau dose is reached. Although the goal is achieving a level in the therapeutic range, whether these ranges can be applied specifically to individuals with dementia is unclear. At the same point, a repeat electrocardiogram should be conducted to look for conduction delays. The patient should be closely monitored for anticholinergic side effects, particularly dry mouth, constipation, blurred vision, and urinary retention.

Monoamine Oxidase Inhibitors

Although the monoamine oxidase inhibitors (MAOIs) are excellent antidepressants, they are infrequently used in the elderly because of their potential to cause debilitating side effects and life-threatening drug–drug and drug–food interactions. Specifically, the combination of MAOIs with other antidepressants; sympathomimetic drugs, including many over-the-counter cold and cough preparations; and tyramine-containing foods can trigger a hypertensive crisis. Given their medical complexity and the use of multiple medications in the typical patient with dementia, the use of MAOIs is not recommended. The MAOIs currently in use are tranylcypromine (Parnate), phenelzine (Nardil), and selegiline (Eldepryl). As Chapter 7 mentions, selegiline is also used to treat Parkinson disease, and it has been studied as a treatment for AD because of the potential antioxidant properties. At doses as high as 10 mg daily, it does not seem to carry a high risk of the dangerous monoamine oxidase side effects.

Psychostimulants

The psychostimulants all consist of forms of amphetamine, and they work by increasing dopaminergic function. They are mainly used to treat attention deficit hyperactivity disorder in children. In adults, they are sometimes used as appetite suppressants, and, in older individuals, they are used to treat apathy, failure to thrive, and late-life depression. The most commonly prescribed stimulant in the elderly is methylphenidate (Ritalin). Two other less commonly prescribed agents are dextroamphetamine (Dexedrine) and pemoline (Cylert). The literature on stimulant use in dementia has been variable, but several studies have found that methylphenidate is beneficial in treating depressive symptoms in older, medically ill patients. Although stimulants were once a popular treatment for these individuals, they have largely been replaced by the SSRIs and bupropion because of the proven efficacy in the treatment of depression, stimulating properties, and relative safety of these latter agents in medically ill patients.

All psychostimulants have a rapid onset of action, short half-lives, and a brief duration of action. For example, onset of action is observed within 1 hour of administering methylphenidate, which has a half-life of 2 to 4 hours; its effects last 3 to 6 hours. Longer-acting preparations have been developed to facilitate duration of action throughout an entire school day for children with attention deficit hyperactivity disorder. In the elderly, dosing is begun at 2.5 to 5 mg in the morning. Look for a positive effect in 2 to 4 hours, and titrate to 5 to 10 mg at morning and noon. Doses given later in the day can lead to insomnia. Pulse and blood pressure should be monitored during the first week of titration, although changes are usually minimal.

The potential side effects include insomnia, anxiety, irritability, anorexia, weight loss, dizziness, headache, and an increased heart rate and blood pressure. Less common, but important, side effects are agitation and psychosis. Stimulants may increase the serum levels of warfarin (Coumadin), anticonvulsants, and TCAs and may potentiate the effects of some narcotics. Although, historically, amphetamines have been drugs of abuse, concern about this is excessive in clinical practice; the potential for physical dependence is extremely low with geriatric dosing.

Treatment Resistance

If an individual has responded partially or not at all after a first-line agent has been started and its dose has been maximized and continued for a 6-week to 8-week trial, several strategies may be considered. First, the clinician should add a behavioral plan or some form of therapeutic contact. Also, he or she should consider whether a move to a more structured setting is warranted. Second, the clinician should switch to another antidepressant, either in the same class (e.g., from one SSRI to aother) or in an entirely different class (e.g., SSRI to mirtazapine). Third, augmenting the antidepressant with another agent should be considered. Frequent combinations include SSRIs plus mirtazapine, venlafaxine, or bupropion; mirtazapine plus venlafaxine; or an SSRI plus an atypical antipsychotic or mood stabilizer. Older strategies, such as adding lithium, beta-blockers, TCAs, or thyroid hormone to an existing antidepressant, can be considered, but the risk of side effects must be weighed carefully. For medication-resistant symptoms, life-threatening depressive symptoms (especially with severe psychosis), or intractable mania, the treatment of choice is electroconvulsive therapy, regardless of age.

BEREAVEMENT

One of the major risk factors for developing depression is grief over the loss of a spouse or loved one. In fact, nearly 25% of widows and widowers present with depression after several months of persistent grief, with men being more severely affected. Even in severe states of dementia, individuals sometimes react to the loss of familiar individuals by demonstrating depressive symptoms. In and of itself, bereavement is not considered a pathologic state, and the form of grieving may vary widely among different cultures. However, when symptoms consistent with a major depressive episode persist beyond 2 months of bereavement, treatment should be considered. Several factors that indicate that a more complicated bereavement has evolved into depression include suicidal ideation, severe guilt, severe functional impairment, and psychosis.

SLEEP DISTURBANCES

Common sleep disorders in late life include sleep apnea, restless legs syndrome, circadian rhythm disorder, periodic limb movement disorder, and rapid eye movement behavior disorder. Sleep disturbances are particularly common in dementia, in which they sometimes manifest as a core symptom of depression. In the latter situation, the symptoms typically include difficulty falling asleep and frequent middle of the night or early morning awakenings. As an individual's depression improves, his or her sleep should improve as well, unless the underlying problem is due more to the dementia or a primary sleep disorder. Unfortunately, these disorders are not always readily diagnosed in individuals with dementia, given the challenges of obtaining an overnight polysomnographic study, especially when the individual has a history of agitation. Sometimes, a physician can make a diagnosis based on the observations of a caregiver or nurse.

The first step in treatment is to improve sleep hygiene in order to facilitate the normal neurophysiologic process of sleep. Sleep hygiene involves both the sleep environment and sleep habits. Several strategies are listed in Table 14.2. These strategies are straightforward, they have no side effects, and they often improve sleep without further intervention. In addition to the focus on sleep hygiene, medications are often needed to restore adequate sleep. Within the setting of depression, a sedating antidepressant, such as mirtazapine or nefazodone, may be sufficient. The clinician should bear in mind, however, that antidepressants, particularly the SSRIs, can sometimes cause insomnia. Otherwise, the mainstay of treating depression-associated sleep disturbances involves the short-term use (10 to 14 days) of a sedative hypnotic agent within the dosing guidelines set by the Omnibus Budget Reconciliation Act. Some of the safest and most efficacious agents are zolpidem (Ambien)

TABLE 14.2. **Strategies for Improving Sleep Hygiene in Dementia**

Avoid stimulants in the afternoon or evening (e.g., coffee, tea, or other drinks or food with caffeine; stimulating antidepressants; dopaminergic agents)

Avoid the use of nicotine and alcohol before sleep

Avoid heavy meals or snacks before bedtime

Maintain consistent, relaxing evening and bedtime routine

Minimize excess lighting and noise during evening and nighttime hours

Avoid waking the patient to dispense medications

Use bed for sleep only; avoid activities in bed, such as reading, watching television

Minimize daytime napping

Maximize daytime exposure to sunlight

Provide adequate daytime activity, including physical exercise

Promote bladder emptying before bedtime and bladder control during sleep

Avoid excess use of diuretics, especially before bedtime

TABLE 14.3. Dosing for Recommended Hypnotics in Dementia

Hypnotic	Starting dose (mg)	Range (mg)
Zolpidem (Ambien)	5	5–10
Zaleplon (Sonata)	5	5–10
Trazodone (Desyrel)	25	25–100
Lorazepam (Ativan)	0.25–0.5	0.25–0.5

and zaleplon (Sonata), as well as low doses of the antidepressant trazodone. When significant anxiety or anxious ruminations associated with poor sleep are present, lorazepam may also be useful. Recommended dosing for these agents appears in Table 14.3. Although melatonin has been studied in the treatment of insomnia, especially that associated with circadian rhythm disturbances, no consensus exists on its efficacy in late life. In the setting of dementia, many geriatric psychiatrists discourage the use of both short-acting benzodiazepines, such as triazolam (Halcion) and alprazolam (Xanax), due to their potential for paradoxical effects and long-acting benzodiazepines, such as temazepam (Restoril) and flurazepam (Dalmane), due to their potential for hangover effects, confusion, and an increased risk of falls. Diphenhydramine should also be avoided in light of its problematic anticholinergic and antihistaminic side effects, including excess sedation, dizziness, and confusion.

 TIP

Sleeping pills are some of the most frequently prescribed medications in the elderly, and they are often taken in excessive doses, for excessive periods, and without proper indication. The clinician must not forget to emphasize sleep hygiene and sleep studies, especially for individuals with resistant symptoms. Sleep apnea is often overlooked, but it can result in significant morbidity and mortality. Daytime function should be examined to gauge the true impact of a sleep disturbance. A patient who complains about insomnia but who is functioning well during the day without excess sedation may actually be receiving adequate sleep.

POOR APPETITE AND/OR FAILURE TO THRIVE

A frequent problem encountered in patients with dementia, especially in those with depression, is poor appetite and weight loss. These problems trigger the following cascade of events: dehydration; malnutrition; decreased renal function; suppressed immune response; worsening medical problems; infection; delayed healing of skin ulcers; and, ultimately, premature death. This precipitous physical and cognitive decline is sometimes referred to as *failure to thrive*. Failure to thrive may range from mild to severe, and it is more common among institutionalized or hospitalized older individuals, especially after they have sustained a hip fracture. Although depression associated with dementia is often an obvious cause of this deadly syndrome, aggressive antidepressant treatment for these individuals is frequently overlooked because their caregivers and clinicians adopt a fatalistic attitude, believing that a terminal phase of dementia has begun. Several strategies may be helpful for poor appetite or failure to thrive.

- Evaluate for difficulty chewing, swallowing (dysphagia), or digesting.
- Evaluate for comorbid medical causes of anorexia, including medications.
- Consider empirical treatment for depression with an antidepressant medication.
- Consider treatment for apathy with a stimulating antidepressant or psychostimulant.
- Consider the use of 15 to 45 mg of mirtazapine daily or 400 to 800 mg of megestrol acetate (Megace) in an oral suspension daily.

As is indicated in the last recommendation, megestrol acetate has been found to improve appetite and to cause weight gain in older individuals with physical wasting or cachexia, whether due to dementia, cancer, or acquired immunodeficiency syndrome.

SUICIDE

The potential for suicidality in depression associated with dementia must be one of the most serious concerns for all clinicians. Older white men, especially those 80 years and older, represent the group at highest risk of suicide in the

United States, with rates that are four to five times greater than those for younger individuals. Older men commit 80% of all suicides in individuals older than 65 years of age, with firearms being the most common method. Depression represents the most significant cause of suicide in this group, but other important risk factors include bereavement over a recent significant loss, living alone, lack of social supports, substance abuse, psychosis, symptoms of panic, severe pain, and chronic illness. Suicide risk should be of particular concern with individuals who are newly diagnosed with dementia and who have some insight into the diagnosis. The risk of suicide decreases in individuals with more severe dementia who lack the cognitive or physical ability to carry out a suicide plan and in residents of long-term care facilities. However, such individuals may instead demonstrate *indirect life-threatening behaviors*, which are defined as repetitive active or passive actions that lead to self-harm and, ultimately, to death. Examples of indirect life-threatening behaviors are refusing food, drink, medications, and medical tests or treatments and unsafe behaviors (e.g., walking into unsafe areas, swallowing foreign bodies or harmful substances).

CLINICAL VIGNETTE

Mr. Singer was an 85-year-old man with a history of moderate dementia, diabetes mellitus, and paranoid delusions. After being moved from his apartment to a nursing home, he began refusing to eat and to take his medications. He also refused to allow the nurses to check his blood glucose. Despite being started on an antidepressant, he rapidly developed dehydration and renal failure, necessitating hospitalization. He subsequently developed pneumonia and died.

Regardless of the stage of dementia, the occurrence of suicidal threats, gestures, attempts, or indirect life-threatening behaviors should prompt immediate clinical assessment, suicide precautions, and the aggressive treatment of depression. Suicide precautions include the removal of sharp or other potentially dangerous objects, safekeeping of medications, and 24-hour monitoring, until a clinician has indicated that the risk has abated. Severe situations should always prompt immediate assessment, followed by hospitalization in a secure psychiatric facility.

APATHY

Overview of Apathy

Apathy is a syndrome characterized by diminished goal-directed activity due to a lack of motivation. In contrast, depression is a disorder of mood, not just motivation. The presence of apathy does not imply an underlying diagnosis of depression, although the two can occur together. Apathy is actually the most common behavioral problem in dementia, as it is seen in 60% to 90% of patients with AD. It is of great importance to caregivers and clinicians because it interferes with patient care and limits their participation in social and therapeutic activities. Apathy can result from strokes or other damage to one or more areas of the brain, including the frontal cortex (especially the dorsolateral regions), thalamus, striatum, and amygdala. Direct damage to the frontal lobes or to subcortical nuclei that have white matter connections to the frontal lobes is perhaps the most common setting in which apathy is seen. Apathy can also result from functional impairment to any of these brain structures, such as that seen in psychiatric disease or as a result of medications or metabolic disturbances. Two of the more common pharmacologic causes are beta-blockers and antipsychotics.

Apathy and depression can seem clinically indistinguishable. Many caregivers complain that their loved one is stubborn or perhaps even depressed because the patient has no interests or motivation, because he or she does not start conversations or answer questions with much detail, or because he or she is less sociable and is unwilling to participate in activities. The caregivers can become overly frustrated and angry with the affected person, causing them to constantly complain and nag. The caregivers do not realize, however, that, when apathy is the cause, no amount of cajoling will motivate the affected person. At that point, clinical diagnosis and treatment become important.

CLINICAL VIGNETTE

Mr. Hoffman, an 84-year-old man with AD, lived with his wife of 40 years. Mrs. Hoffman was relatively healthy and physically fit, and she enjoyed socializing with her friends and engaging in various activities and community involvements. She told her physician that she was frustrated with her husband because he sat quietly all day in front of the television and rarely spoke to her. She tried to take him to a day program, but he did not actively participate. She brought him to social events, but he would not engage in any meaningful conversation with friends. She often found him sitting somewhat contentedly in his chair, staring out the window. She was angry that he would not try to help himself and feared that he might be severely depressed.

Several clinical keys can help to answer the question of whether Mr. Hoffman is depressed or merely apathetic. When the clinician is evaluating a person's recent psychiatric history, he or she should look for some of the following symptoms that are common to depression but rare with apathy: suicidal ideation, somatic complaints, anxious or depressive ruminations, and hallucinations or delusions. Affect also can differentiate the two states—in depression, affect may appear as overtly sad or depressed, weepy, labile, irritable, angry, or anxious, whereas, in apathy, affect tends to be placid or neutral, flat, and blunted. During the mental status examination, depressed individuals with dementia may become upset, impatient, or irritable with the questioning, sometimes refusing to answer. Individuals with apathy, conversely, often sit and stare during the mental status examination, demonstrating minimal spontaneous speech and motor movements. Responses to questions often consist only of one or two words, and even persistent questioning will not evoke more detail. The apathetic individual rarely confabulates because motivation is required for that.

Treatment of Apathy

Treatment of a reversible cause of apathy often results in clinical improvement. Apathy due to the specific brain damage associated with the dementia is more difficult to treat, and it responds poorly to environmental, behavioral, or psychotherapeutic intervention. The individual simply does not have enough motivation to engage in such therapy. Instead, psychopharmacologic treatment must be used to attempt some improvement. Stimulating antidepressants, such as bupropion or the SSRIs, are usually the treatment of choice, particularly bupropion because of its dopaminergic properties. Psychostimulants can also be used because they may increase motivation and activity level in some individuals.

Acetylcholinesterase (AChE) inhibitors are commonly prescribed for individuals with apathy, although they are used less to treat the apathy and more to treat the underlying dementia. Clinical trials indicate, however, that AChE inhibitor therapy may improve symptoms of apathy, as well as cognition and function. Strictly dopaminergic agents, including bromocriptine (Parlodel), amantadine (Symmetrel), and pergolide (Permax), are used infrequently because of the lack of convincing evidence of their efficacy and their multiple potential side effects (e.g., hypotension, dry mouth, nausea and vomiting, sleep disruptions, psychosis).

PSYCHOSOCIAL ISSUES IN DEMENTIA CARE

Caring for the Caregiver

Essential Concepts
- Caregivers are the core of dementia care. Wives, daughters, and daughters-in-law comprise 90% of caregivers.
- *Caregiver burden* refers to the physical, emotional, and financial toll of caregiving. This includes increased rates of depression, illness, and mortality.
- Despite the enormous burden of caregiving, ways to decrease stress and improve caregiving skills are numerous.

The main focus of nearly every chapter in this book is on the individual with dementia. However, emphasizing the necessity of dementia workup, diagnosis, and treatment without discussing a critical component—the caregiver—would be misleading. Every individual with dementia requires some degree of assistance with daily living. The degree of assistance varies, depending on the type and stage of dementia, but all individuals with a progressive dementia, such as Alzheimer disease (AD), eventually require total care. The estimated number of individuals with dementia in the United States is five million, and nearly twice that number of individuals serve as informal caregivers. These caregivers assume enormous responsibility and burdens, day in and day out for years, particularly when they are caring for someone at home. They must spend time with the affected individual preparing meals, ensuring adequate hygiene, administering medications, taking them to places and appointments, engaging them in activities, monitoring their whereabouts and safety, and so on. Such caregiving is more than a full-time job, and the burden is often physically and emotionally draining, exacting a toll in terms of the caregiver's health and even his or her life span. The term *caregiver burden* has been widely used to describe the resulting physical, emotional, and financial tolls. Even after an individual is placed in a long-term care institution and the burden of caregiving shifts to a larger group of individuals, the primary caregiver can be left with feelings of guilt, sadness, and depression, in addition to the ongoing struggle of watching a loved one succumb to a tragic illness. This chapter describes these caregivers and the incredible burden that they face, and it provides numerous tips on how the clinician can help them cope with dementia and optimize dementia care.

CLINICAL VIGNETTE

Interview with a Caregiver

The following interview is based on a social worker's interview of the 76-year-old wife of Mr. Arden, a 78-year-old man with a 6-year history of AD. He had lived at home with Mrs. Arden until 4 months ago, when he was admitted to a long-term care facility. Mrs. Arden continues to live at home, and she visits him 5 or 6 days a week (SW, social worker; Mrs. A., Mrs. Arden/caregiver).

SW: *Tell me what it was like when your husband developed Alzheimer disease.*

Mrs. A: *It was just terrible. At first, he began to forget to do things around the house, but then he began wandering off. We were once on a vacation in Las Vegas, and I told him to wait by the bathroom in the casino while I went in. He wandered off, and I couldn't find him for hours, even with the help of the police. It was a ruined vacation.*

SW: *How were you able to care for him?*

Mrs. A: *In the early stages, I could leave him alone for short periods of time. After the wandering incident, however, I had to stay with him 24 hours a day. My daughter sometimes came over to help, but I felt guilty every time I left the house. I would try to go out to lunch with a girlfriend, but then I would get this unsettling guilty feeling, like I was abandoning him. I never really enjoyed time away, although it did help. As he got worse, I had to hire a girl to come in and bathe him several times a week. He would fight me when I tried to shave him, and once he gave me a black eye. He would go to the bathroom in his pants but refuse to let me change him. The worst was when he would wake up at night and wander around the house, sometimes making a racket in the kitchen. He fell several times, once breaking his arm. I slept with one eye open and was exhausted most days. Finally, my daughter said that enough was enough.*

SW: *Since he was admitted to the nursing home, have things been better?*

Mrs. A: *Things are better because I can finally sleep at night. It is easier physically, but I still feel badly emotionally. I feel* *guilty when I'm not here. He always asked me never to put him away, and now…(crying)…I can't believe what life has dealt us. We've been married 55 years. I try to come every day. I make sure that he is taken care of and I help feed him. He used to be such a fun, vibrant person, but now he is just a shell. He doesn't speak any more—that is one of the toughest things—I can't talk with him.*

Mrs. Arden describes many common themes for caregivers, including the following: endless hours of exhausting tasks, episodes of frightening and humiliating behavioral disturbances, and strong feelings of guilt and grief that last for years. Caregivers often suffer in silence, feeling too embarrassed or too isolated to confide in others, including clinicians, until the situation becomes unbearable.

CAREGIVERS AND CAREGIVER BURDEN

In the setting of dementia, a caregiver is any individual who assumes the primary responsibility of caring for an individual with dementia. One estimate has indicated that 70% to 80% of all individuals with dementia are cared for at home, with most of the care being provided by family members. Furthermore, 80% to 90% of all caregivers are estimated to be women, and 40% to 50%, to be spouses. Daughters and daughters-in-law account for another 40% of caregivers, while sons and other individuals account for less than 10%. On average, home caregivers spend as many as 70 hours a week assisting an individual with moderate to severe dementia.

As has been noted, the term *burden* reflects the negative impact of caregiving on both the individual's physical and emotional functioning and his or her financial resources. The physical toll is clear—caregivers have higher rates of medical illness and slower recovery times, they make significantly more physician visits, they use more prescription drugs, and they have a higher mortality rate. Caregivers do not fare any better emotionally, with increased rates of depression, anxiety, exhaustion, and sleep and appetite problems, as well as greater use of psychotropic medications. An estimated 20% to 50% of caregivers experience depression, reflecting a two to three times greater risk than that seen in the general population. Not surprisingly, caregivers who are under stress lose more days of work and tend to be less productive. The burden on the part of the caregivers has also been associated with increased stress and behavioral problems in the individual with dementia, resulting in a greater likelihood of eventual long-term care placement.

The financial toll is significant. Caregivers spend an estimated $5,800 yearly for unreimbursable services and supplies for the individual with dementia, a figure that increases to more than $10,000 for individuals with more severe dementia. In addition, caregivers can face agonizing decisions when they are contemplating nursing home placement for the individual with dementia because it can quickly deplete their life savings.

 KEY POINT

Research has found that the single most important factor that increases burden is the lack of *respite time*. This includes time for private activities, errands, and social engagements and simply time away from their caregiving responsibilities.

ASSESSMENT OF BURDEN

Every dementia workup and all follow-up visits with an individual with dementia should include attention to the caregiver, with questions about how he or she is coping with his or her loved one's illness and whether he or she has help. Interviewing the caregiver alone to allow him or her to be more open without worrying about upsetting the loved one is sometimes wise. Signs of caregiver stress include feelings of exhaustion, guilt, anger, and anxiety; social withdrawal and isolation; impaired sleep and concentration; increased health problems; and a decline in caregiving, which sometimes is reflected in the condition of the individual with dementia. Two brief measures for caregiver burden are the Burden Interview and the Screen for Caregiver Burden. (See the "Suggested Readings" section of this text for references for these tools.) A practical "mini" burden interview can be found on Pocket Card D.1 in Appendix D. Regardless of the outward signs, the caregiver's perceived burden is ultimately the most important factor. Caregivers who perceive themselves as being under more stress tend to fare worse; caregivers with positive perceptions who are bolstered by active coping styles, family support, and spirituality do better.

 TIP

If a caregiver admits to feelings of depression, hopelessness, or helplessness or to feeling overwhelmed, the clinician should *always* inquire about suicidal and homicidal thoughts. The intensity of the burden can be so overwhelming for some caregivers that they consider ending their own life and the life of the individual with dementia. Suicide-homicides are a small but growing problem; they are more common in elderly couples in which the husband is the primary caregiver. Caregiver risk factors for suicide–homicide include social isolation, higher socioeconomic status, medical problems, depression, and a controlling personality.

CONFLICT WITH CAREGIVERS

A particular subset of caregivers can be difficult to assess and help, and this group may prove disruptive to the doctor–patient relationship and to long-term care. Such caregivers struggle with both informal and formal supports, including their friends and family, professionals, and staff members at supportive agencies, programs, and institutions. These struggles often stem from inflexible or even pathologic coping styles, behavioral patterns, or personalities. They are fueled by the stress and strong emotions inherent to the caregiver role. For example, a caregiver may feel deep anger at his or her loved one for being ill, but, instead, he or she directs it at those trying to help. He or she may feel inadequate as a caregiver or guilty about having to place the loved one in an institution, and he or she then projects these feelings onto external supports. The resulting anger, accusations, and demands can create turmoil in the caregiving setting, leaving the caregiver isolated from those who want to help.

CLINICAL VIGNETTE

Mr. Robins is a retired physician who visits his wife daily at the nursing home and spends 5 to 6 hours helping to care for her. His obsessive-compulsive personality drives him to keep meticulous records of his wife's care, down to the daily temperature readings and bowel movement characteristics. He frequently berates staff members for minor mistakes and demands that custodial staff and nursing aides be available whenever he calls. He has had numerous fights with both the administrative and clinical staff because he tries to dictate details of his wife's care.

When a clinician has had a difficult encounter with a caregiver, he or she should not jump to "diagnose" the caregiver or to assign blame to him or her. Instead, the clinician must recognize the role of clinical staff or other factors that may be causing part of the problem. Remaining an empathic and open listener to the caregiver and providing timely and honest communication are essential. At the same time, however, the clinician may need to educate the caregiver on the limits of his or her own role and to provide the caregiver with relevant referrals to other professionals. The clinician should always consider involving other team members whose specialties may lend themselves to specific aspects of the conflict. In institutions, the administrative and legal staff may need to be involved.

CARING FOR THE CAREGIVER

The following basic rules for any clinician to help caregivers to cope with their situation and reduce stress are simple: be available and supportive; listen; communicate; and guide them to available resources. The clinician must bear in mind the fact that caregivers are undergoing a tremendous change in their lives, having to shift their previous roles and responsibilities to take on difficult new tasks. For example, the spouse of the adult patient with dementia finds himself or herself assuming responsibilities that are reminiscent of past parenting with young children, including constant monitoring, toileting, feeding, and bathing. Gender roles can be reversed as a husband or wife has to assume the unfamiliar tasks once handled by the spouse, such as managing household finances, routine cleaning and maintenance of the home and yard, and grocery shopping. In addition, a spouse may lose his or her main source of communication and support.

Furthermore, the previous patterns of intimacy and sexuality with the loved one often decline and eventually cease, leaving the caregiver without a partner for his or her intimate needs. An older caregiver also must struggle to maintain adequate levels of energy, enthusiasm, and concentration for meeting the needs of his or her loved one, despite being beset by his or her own physical and emotional problems.

Adult children who serve as caregivers face similar physical and emotional demands, but their perspective is different. Many women, in particular, are faced with the dual roles of caring both for children and teenagers and for an aged parent with dementia, leaving little time for other interests, a situation that has led to them being aptly described by the term "sandwich generation." The adult children also face the emotional burden of having to reverse the parent–child role, especially when they are dealing with toileting, bathing, and behavioral problems with a parent. Sons who have relied on their wives to provide most of the hands-on child care in their own household may be particularly perplexed and frustrated by such caregiving; they may instead defer the assumption of many responsibilities to a sister, wife, or hired aide.

Grief, loss, confusion, anger, frustration, all of which are emotional reactions to seeing a loved one suffer from dementia, can trigger previous unresolved feelings toward, or conflicts with, the individual with dementia. The reactions of caregivers vary widely, and they are unpredictable. Some caregivers act out with inappropriate and excessive behaviors, accounting for some of the reactions of difficult caregivers that were described earlier. A son or daughter who never got much attention from the parent may now feel even angrier as the dementia robs them of a chance to make up for lost time, or he or she may plunge into caregiving with excessive zeal to try to heal this emotional wound. Previously abusive parents who now have dementia may be neglected by family members who feel freed of their domination or who seek "revenge" for years of abuse. However, most individuals who are unable to cope with past unresolved conflicts benefit from support groups and therapy. The clinician's understanding of these dynamics helps him or her to provide the best care and to select the most relevant resources.

KEY STRATEGIES: THE SIX Es

With all of these factors in mind, the important strategies for helping caregivers best meet the care demands of an individual with dementia are represented by the mnemonic *the Six Es* as follows:

- **Educate** caregivers about the diagnosis, disease course, and available resources;
- **Empower** the strengths of the caregiver and the abilities of the patient with dementia;
- **Environmental** comfort, stimulation, and safety organize caregiving, protect the individual with dementia, and optimize his or her course;
- **Engage** both caregivers and patients in stimulating, comfortable, and structured activities;
- **Energize** the ability to be a good caregiver by taking care of his or her needs and providing respite time;
- **End points** are long-term care placement and hospice care; foster realistic attitudes and be proactive toward these inevitabilities without engaging in excessive pessimism.

Educate

Fear and confusion are two of the greatest barriers for caregivers, and each can take a significant toll. Most caregivers do not fully understand the exact diagnosis and course of the disease, and, thus, they have difficulty understanding and making decisions about events that take place along the way. Clinicians have the responsibility of reviewing all this information with caregivers. They must teach them what to expect along the way without unduly frightening them and guide them toward organizations, websites, readings, and other resources that can help. Many of these are listed at the end of this chapter.

Empower

Although clinicians spend so much time focusing on the caregiver burden, they must always keep in mind the wellspring of caregiver strengths that carry them from day to day. These strengths are their physical and psychologic abilities, their intellectual skills, their social supports, their financial resources, and their spiritual or religious inclinations. Clinicians can help caregivers recognize and optimize their strengths. Table 15.1 lists a variety of tips to help empower caregivers in taking an active role in enhancing dementia care.

TABLE 15.1. Tips on Enhancing Dementia Care

Enhance communication
  Use simple, direct language, and repeat it as needed
  Use friendly and engaging nonverbal cues (e.g., eye contact, smiles, touches)
  Compensate for sensory limitations (e.g., glasses, hearing aids)
  Limit distractions, such as excessive noise or commotion
Enhance memory
  Provide daily orientation with large-print calendars and lists
  Label drawers, closets, and so on with explanatory words or pictures
  Post a list of important phone contacts near the phone
  Always introduce visitors by name and relationship
Enhance daily caregiving
  Structure daily caregiving but allow some flexibility
  Break up caregiving into easier, quicker, and more tolerable tasks
  Get assistance from aides, nurses, friends, and family
  Prepare the room and needed accessories ahead of time
  Encourage the dementia patient to exercise as much control as possible
  Ensure dignity and privacy during bathing, toileting, grooming, and dressing

Environment

An assessment of the caregiving environment is outlined in Chapter 3, which focuses on identifying potentially unsafe situations. The home environment can be adapted to optimize the safety and function of the individual with dementia. Potentially hazardous substances, medications, and items such as power tools and firearms should be locked away, and exits and stairs should be safeguarded to prevent an individual with dementia from wandering away from the house. The Alzheimer's Association sponsors a program called *Safe Return* that assists in the event that an individual with dementia gets lost outside the home (call 1-800-272-3900 to register a person). To improve ambulation and minimize the risk of falls, the environment can be enhanced by removing excess furniture and clutter and installing proper lighting, nonslip rugs and mats, and assist bars in the bathroom. Caregivers should keep up the regular maintenance of the home, yard, car, major appliances, and utilities, and they should have a list of repair services and emergency contacts.

The most unsafe situation is that of an individual with dementia who is living alone without sufficient monitoring and assistance. When a situation involving compromised safety, neglect, abuse, or exploitation is suspected, necessary interventions may include consultation with a social worker or case manager and contacting the local agency that investigates potential abuse. Sometimes, the police must be contacted when an imminent threat is suspected.

Engage

Even in later stages of progressive dementia, individuals retain the ability to respond to sensory stimulation in positive ways. At any stage in dementia, such stimulation can be critical to the individual with dementia maintaining engagement with his or her surrounding world, attachment to loved ones, a sense of identity and integrity, and dignity. For caregivers and family, the engagement of the individual with dementia in the world around him or her is a healthy and productive approach to dementia. Unfortunately, family members sometimes react out of depression, anger, guilt, disgust, and grief and disengage from the individual with dementia, either actively through staying away or passively by visiting in body but not in mind or spirit. Caregivers who see no meaning to the life of a person with dementia may discourage visits from loved ones, or the loved ones may feel unsure about what to do during visits other than sit and count the minutes.

A counterpoint to these attitudes is the approach that emphasizes in every stage of dementia that individuals with dementia retain engageable strengths. The clinician should ask caregivers the following questions about the individual with dementia:

- What are they still able to do at their current stage?
- What did they love to do earlier in life?
- What held great meaning for them?
- Are cultural or religious items, rituals, foods, music, languages, or individuals that held great meaning for them present?
- What form of sensory stimulation can they still enjoy?

The clinician should make a list of every capability that he or she can generate from these questions as the first step toward maintaining vital engagement. In long-term care facilities, the social workers and recreational therapists rely on these strengths to plan appropriate activities and programs. For individuals with dementia who are living at home, caregivers must find resources in the community to help. Such resources may include programs at religious or cultural centers and houses of worship, senior centers, adult day care programs, support groups, and friendly visitor programs. Table 15.2 contains a list of suggested activities. Several of the books listed at the end of the chapter also contain suggestions.

Children and teenagers who have a loved one suffering from dementia may sometimes react to the situation with confusion, fear, and anger. They may not understand why their grandparent forgets things, does not recognize them at times, or acts dif-

TABLE 15.2. Suggested Activities with a Dementia Patient

Sensory stimulation
    Prepare and eat a favorite food together
    Take a walk through a serene garden or park
    Hand massage with oils or lotion
    Hugging, holding hands
    Bring soft objects and stuffed animals to hold
    Listen to music
Reminiscing
    Look at old photograph albums together
    Listen to music from an earlier period in the patient's life
    Ask about early memories that may be retained
    Visit an old friend
    Converse in a first language together
Intergenerational activities with children, grandchildren, and
    great-grandchildren
    Look at old photographs and take new ones
    Decorate room, wheelchair, and/or walker together
    Participate in arts and crafts
    Watch movies together
    Plant something that will grow, continually reminding children of
      the visit
Physical activities
    Do household chores together
    Engage in mild exercise, such as stretching or walks
    Participate in simple sports (fishing, horseshoes, catching soft
      ball)
Religious/spiritual activities
    Attend religious service together
    Have the clergy visit
    Read religious texts and pray together
    Celebrate holidays and conduct rituals together

ferently. They may fear that they or their parents will get dementia, or they may be afraid of particular behaviors, especially when the individual displays psychosis or agitation. They may be angry if the affected person or the caregiver spends less time with them. Sometimes, these reactions are clearly stated; at other times, they are acted out indirectly, perhaps at school or with friends. The clinician should recognize the importance of both identifying these reactions and helping the family to engage children and teenagers with their loved one with dementia. The clinician should also educate young persons, at their level of understanding, about dementia. He or she should use examples rather than technical descriptions in discussing dementia with young persons, should inquire about their feelings, and should find constructive ways for these to be expressed. The caregiver should not expect, nor ask, them to help with caregiving responsibilities, especially bathing and hygiene. If they offer to help with some tasks, the caregiver should find easy, nonthreatening things for them to do with the person with dementia, such as simple physical activity or games, arts and crafts, and reminiscing (Table 15.2).

CLINICAL VIGNETTE

Mrs. Pierre, a 78-year-old Haitian woman, was admitted to a nursing home due to severe dementia and associated agitation at home. In the first month, she continued to be agitated, and she often refused to eat. The staff had difficulty understanding her because she only spoke Creole. Her three daughters were distraught over her condition, and they felt guilty and angry about putting her in the facility. The social worker, Mrs. Tressler, convened a family meeting and asked them to tell her about their mother. Words and tears flowed for more than an hour as the Pierre family described a strong matriarch who had brought them from Haiti to the United States and had worked several jobs to put them all through school. They described her loves as preparing Haitian foods, sewing, and spending time with their young children. Mrs. Tressler asked the family to work with the dietitian to bring in some of Mrs. Pierre's favorite foods. They arranged for a Creole-speaking aide to visit her daily and to bring her to arts and crafts for sewing. The daughters also were encouraged to visit and to bring along the grandchildren on a regular basis. Mrs. Pierre reacted well to these changes and quickly regained the lost weight.

Energize

Caregivers need to take care of themselves and to reenergize on a regular basis to avoid burn out. One of the best ways to reenergize is simply to have a break from caregiving to run errands and to spend time socially with friends. Another way is going on short trips, perhaps to visit family in other parts of the country. Life cannot stop entirely for the caregiver; otherwise, he or she is guaranteed to suffer from excess burden that ultimately will impair his or her caregiving ability. Caregivers should be encouraged to attend concerts, to eat out, to have beauty treatments, and to engage in relaxing and aesthetically pleasing activities. Caregivers should also tend to their own physical and mental health by engaging in exercise, maintaining a healthy diet, and getting adequate sleep. Religious and spiritual connections can also help.

SEXUALITY IN DEMENTIA

Despite a diagnosis of dementia, sexuality may continue to be an important factor in the lives of many individuals and their partners. For these couples, sexual intimacy can provide a nonverbal means of communication and connection. As dementia progresses into the more severe states, however, the ability to initiate sexual activity, to provide consent, and to sustain performance may become impaired. Caregivers may face other difficulties as well, including sexually aggressive or inappropriate behaviors (see Chapters 12 and 13) and ethical issues regarding extramarital relationships and competency to consent to sexual activity. Despite the centrality of all of these issues for caregivers, health care professionals often fail to inquire about them.

Dementia can affect sexuality in several ways. In general, research indicates that sexual activity is decreased by more than 50% in couples with a partner with Alzheimer disease. Many possible explanations for this exist. Caregivers may be turned off and may have less sexual desire for a partner with dementia who does not always recognize them, who is less physically attractive (i.e., due to poor hygiene, incontinence, loss of motor or language functions), or who requests sex repeatedly because he or she cannot remember when they last had it. Caregivers may be confused by their conflicting feelings of love and fidelity for their spouse with dementia and guilt over their desires for extramarital intimacy. The depression experienced by both caregivers and patients with dementia can also be associated with a loss of sexual desire. The dementia process itself may be a culprit because the cognitive impairment may reduce the individual's attentional capacity during sex, as well as the ability to initiate and sequence components of lovemaking. Despite all of these factors, sexual dysfunction is not the rule in dementia, and sexual desire may remain strong or it may even increase as previously held inhibitions are reduced by cognitive impairment.

When assessing a couple in which one partner has dementia, clinicians should inquire about sexual problems, such as loss of desire, erectile dysfunction, or other problems that interfere with lovemaking. The clinician should not let his or her own discomfort in discussing sexual topics get in the way of helping the couple. The following simple recommendations can help many couples with sexual problems.

- Shift the focus from sexual intercourse to physical intimacy and foreplay.
- Rule out causes of sexual dysfunction, such as medical problems or medications.
- Encourage gynecologic or urologic consultation when necessary.

In long-term care facilities, the staff has the responsibility of ensuring privacy for conjugal visits. With more severe states of dementia, however, the cognitively intact partner may question whether the patient with dementia retains the capacity to consent to sexual activity. The issue of an individual's capacity to consent to sex is covered in Chapter 16.

END POINTS

A major endpoint occurs in the later stages of dementia when the individual is no longer able to live in his or her current environment, so he or she must be placed in a more structured one. Although this usually means a move from his or her home to a long-term care facility, it can also refer to moves from an independent to an assisted-living facility or from an open to a closed dementia or behavioral unit within a facility. How does the clinician know when the patient has reached an end point with respect to the environment? Signs may include the following:

- Recurrent accidents or behavioral problems by the patient with dementia;
- Caregiver who is physically or psychologically incapacitated;
- An environment that is always unsafe or unkempt;
- A patient with dementia who is being neglected or abused;
- A caregiver who is not able to meet the needs of the patient.

Caregivers often agonize over nursing home placement because of a view that nursing homes are unpleasant and impersonal places that warehouse elders in their remaining days, or they may object to a move to a more structured unit because they view its residents as "more impaired" than their loved one or because they see the move as a harbinger of impending death. Patients often resist moving for similar reasons. Being proactive is always better because it allows the caregiver more time to explore possibilities and to make a choice without a crisis looming.

CLINICAL VIGNETTE

Mrs. Lubin, an 89-year-old woman with worsening memory impairment and a long history of dementia, lived in an assisted-living facility. Because of her failing cognition, increased anxiety, and frequent crying episodes in the dining hall, the staff advised the family to move her to their dementia floor. When Mrs. Lubin was informed about this plan, she carried on for days, crying, pleading with staff, and threatening to kill herself. When the day of the move arrived, she went along passively. She adjusted nicely to the new unit, and she was less anxious and tearful.

Meeting Resistance

When the clinician is advising a family and patient that a move is necessary, he or she must gauge their readiness for the decision. The clinician should broach the topic and discuss the pros and cons without insisting on a course of action, as the caregivers always appreciate a calm, nonpressured discussion. When the clinician meets resistance, he or she should ask the caregivers to explore alternative ways to increase structure and support in the existing environment. Sometimes, additional resources, such as visiting nurses, aides, or companions, can improve the situation and buy the caregiver time. Cognition, function, and behavior in the existing environment should be optimized through appropriate treatment of any underlying medical and psychiatric problems. When problems persist, however, the clinician should advise the caregivers to visit several potential facilities to learn about their options. He or she may suggest a transitional admission to a hospital when this is appropriate, such as when the individual with dementia has significant behavioral problems that warrant a geriatric psychiatry evaluation before placement can even be considered. As long as the patient has no imminent risk of harm, however, the clinician can do little, short of making repeated recommendations. Some patients and families have to fail on the outside and unfortunately to suffer consequences, such as injury or hospitalization, before they realize that the current situation is not safe.

Easing the Transition to Long-Term Care

To smooth the process of admission to a long-term care facility, the clinician should encourage the caregivers to prepare the person and the new environment for the move. This may include making visits ahead of time, speaking with staff about the person's background and special needs, and preparing the new room ahead of time with photographs, personal items, and other touches of home and comfort (e.g., a colorful quilt, a working radio and television). Residents or caregivers should not bring in heirlooms or expensive or irreplaceable items whose damage or disappearance may devastate them. Instead, they should bring in copies of old photographs, costume jewelry, and inexpensive appliances that can easily be replaced. Caregivers should plan to spend time with the individual on the day of admission, and friends and family should be encouraged to call or to visit frequently. They should make personal contact with the nursing and social work staff and should supply them with an accurate medical and psychiatric history and medication lists.

The first few weeks are often difficult for the affected individual, and extra care and attention are critical; this sometimes requires the assistance of part-time private duty aides.

The stereotype of institutions as cold, impersonal places is usually false; a lot of warmth and caring are seen and many enriching activities take place daily in most long-term care facilities. Family involvement is always welcome, and it adds to the sense of community.

The Final End Point: Hospice and Palliative Care

The final end point occurs when an individual with a progressive dementia enters a terminal state, which is usually characterized by a severe decline in function in which the individual can no longer walk, swallow, or communicate verbally. Ethical issues, such as advance directives, tube feeding, and *do not resuscitate* status, are discussed in Chapter 16. From the standpoint of both the caregiver and palliative care, the goal is to maximize the comfort of the patient in a dignified and compassionate way. Hospice care in dementia involves the control and palliation of pain and discomfort for the patient and counseling and spiritual guidance for both the patient and caregiver. This does not mean that anything is done to hasten the patient's death, but it does recognize the limitations of care, the inevitability of death, and the value of comfort and dignity. Several resources on hospice care are listed at the end of the chapter

---

 KEY POINT

Even in severe stages of dementia, affected individuals are often still capable of receiving and giving affection, warmth, and personal communication. Caregivers are sometimes the best teachers for clinicians with respect to this point as they persist in providing love and affection for individuals who seem incapable of engaging with it. The health care profession demands that we persist in our efforts to treat individuals with dementia in a compassionate and dignified manner throughout the entire progression of disease.

CAREGIVER RESOURCES

All the following organizations and websites can provide information, resources, and referrals for caregivers and individuals with dementia.

Organizations

Alzheimer's Association: phone, (800) 272-3900; website, http://www.alz.org

Alzheimer's Disease Education and Referral Center: phone, (800) 438-4380; website, http://www.alzheimers.org

American Health Assistance Foundation (AHAF): phone, (800) 437-2423; website, http://www.ahaf.org

American Association for Geriatric Psychiatry: phone, (301) 654-7850; website, http://www.aagponline.org

Children of Aging Parents: phone, (800) 227-7294; website, http://www.caps4caregivers.org

National Association for Home Care: phone, (202) 547-7424; website, http://www.nahc.org

National Association of Area Agencies on Aging: phone, (202) 296-8130; website, http://www.n4a.org

National Family Caregivers Association: phone, (800) 896-3650; website, http://www.nfcacares.org

National Hospice and Palliative Care Organization: phone, (800) 658-8898; hospice helpline and locator, (703) 837-1500; websites, http://www.nhpco.org or http://www.hospiceinfo.org

Senior Companion Program: phone, (800) 424-8867; website, http://www.seniorcorps.org/joining/scp/

Well Spouse Foundation: phone, (800) 838-8815; website, http://www.wellspouse.org

Ageless Design: a website with articles, tips, news, links, and an online store for dementia-related books and products; http://www.agelessdesign.com

Elderweb: a website for caregivers to research home and long-term care, legal and financial issues, housing options, and medical issues; http://www.elderweb.com

Eldercare Locator: a nationwide, directory assistance service that links up older caregivers with local supports and resources; phone, (800) 677-1116

Books for Caregivers

Bell V, Troxel D. *The best friends approach to Alzheimer's care.* Baltimore: Health Professions Press, 1997.

Bridges BJ, Temairik J. *Therapeutic caregiving: a practical guide for caregivers of persons with Alzheimer's and other dementia causing diseases.* Mill Creek, WA: BJB Publishing, 1998.

Fitzray BJ. *Alzheimer's activities: hundreds of activities for men and women with Alzheimer's disease and related disorders.* Windsor, CA: Rayve Productions, 2001.

Mace NL, Rabins PV. *The 36-hour day: revised edition. A family guide to caring for persons with Alzheimer's disease, related dementing illness, and memory loss in later life.* Baltimore: John Hopkins University Press, 1999.

Powell L. *Alzheimer's disease: a guide for families and caregivers,* 3rd ed. Cambridge, MA: Perseus Publishing, 2002.

Strauss CJ. *Talking to Alzheimer's: simple ways to connect when you visit a family member or friend.* Oakland, CA: New Harbinger Publications, 2002.

Warner ML. *The complete guide to Alzheimer's-proofing your home,* rev. ed. West Lafayette, IN: Purdue University Press, 2000.

Legal and Ethical Issues

Essential Concepts
- Legal and ethical issues arise when an individual with dementia is no longer able to make rational decisions regarding various aspects of his or her life.
- The underlying principles of ethics that guide decision making include autonomy, beneficence, justice, and confidentiality.
- Key legal and ethical issues associated with dementia include the determination of competency, diagnostic truth telling, genetic testing, informed consent and participation in research, driving, the use of restraints, sexual relationships, advance directives, and end-of-life care.
- The discussion of any legal and ethical issue in dementia care must begin with a knowledge of the individual's degree of cognitive and functional impairment and the availability of surrogate decision makers.

From the very first signs and symptoms of dementia, clinicians, caregivers, and patients must face unique and important legal and ethical issues. These issues arise because the disease, in whatever form it takes, impairs an individual's capacity to make decisions and to function independently. End-of-life issues, in particular, have become more prominent and more complex in the past few decades because the practice of medicine has increasingly achieved the ability to prolong the lives of individuals with dementia despite their severe physical and mental incapacity. The ability of a clinician to understand these issues and to intervene effectively and appropriately depends on a thorough assessment that has led to the diagnosis of dementia and its stage; an awareness of the religious, cultural, and philosophic factors that influence decision making for both the patient and family; and personal involvement with the family and other surrogate decision makers.

PRINCIPLES OF ETHICS

Several of the following fundamental principles of ethics underlie this chapter:

Autonomy or self-determination: to the extent possible, individuals have the right to make their own decisions and to have them respected by others.

Beneficence: clinicians have a responsibility to act for the good of the patient. The corollary to beneficence is non-maleficence, or do no harm to the patient.

Justice: clinicians and health care institutions should treat patients fairly when making decisions about care and allocation of resources.

Confidentiality: clinicians have a responsibility to ensure the integrity and confidentiality of all medical records and communication. This principle has received increased attention in the past few years as a result of the privacy provisions for health care contained in the Health Insurance Portability and Accountability Act, or HIPAA, enacted in 1996.

Several essential *virtues* that clinicians should possess that help in implementing and safeguarding these principles are honesty, empathy, respect for dignity, discretion, and a commitment to mutual communication.

CAPACITY AND COMPETENCE

Capacity is the clinical term for an individual's relative cognitive ability to understand or do something, while *competency* refers to a judge's determination of this ability in an individual. Although the two terms are often used interchangeably, their legal distinction should be understood. Both terms should always be invoked with respect to a specific purpose, including the following:

- Making health care decisions (e.g., seeking or refusing treatment, enrolling in research);
- Making financial or estate decisions (e.g., managing property, giving gifts of money, making a will);
- Living independently and managing personal obligations (e.g., choosing one's own residence, feeding and clothing oneself, taking medications, driving, voting);
- Participating in legal proceedings (e.g., entering into a contract, suing or being sued, standing trial or testifying at one, serving on a jury, marrying).

All individuals are assumed competent unless they are proven otherwise, and a diagnosis of dementia does not automatically imply that someone is incompetent. An individual may retain capacity in one sphere but not in another. Struggles ensue when a clinician, caregiver, or another involved party questions an individual's mental competency, thus prompting further investigation. The clinician must bear in mind, however, that, even with a diagnosis of dementia, individuals can be competent yet still be indecisive or resistant to help, and they can make bad decisions. Sorting through these various possibilities and making a determination of an individual's decision-making ability is the first step in all legal and ethical questions.

Both capacity and competency require that an individual's ability to make his or her own decisions includes the following features:

- Understanding or knowledge of the relevant facts involved in the decision;
- Appreciation of the fact that he or she has a choice, what the consequences of different choices could be (i.e., risks and benefits), and the significance of various facts;
- Ability to think rationally about the choices and to consider, compare, and weigh facts and options in an organized manner;
- Ability to make and express a decision in actuality.

All of these abilities must be present and brought to bear on a specific domain in a consistent manner. A person who can weigh choices one day but not the next cannot consistently make competent decisions. However, an individual could have the capacity to think about and to express a choice about giving a gift to someone but not to drive safely or to serve on a jury. Similarly, an individual may have a limited ability to make choices (e.g., to whom to give a gift of money), but he or she may rely on others to help clarify and implement the decision (e.g., how much money to give and in what manner).

A determination of capacity occurs informally all the time, as clinicians advise patients and their families on what they can or cannot do, with variable compliance. An outline for a formal capacity evaluation is given in Table 16.1. A legal determination of competence can only be decided by a judge, a determination that is based, in part, on the clinician's assessment of mental capacity. If someone is found incompetent in one or more areas, he or she is assigned a surrogate to make decisions for him or her. Depending on the state, various legal terms are used for this surrogate decision maker,

TABLE 16.1. Competency Evaluation in Dementia

---

1. Obtain psychiatric and medical history from the patient and the informants.
2. Conduct a mental status examination.
3. Query the patient with respect to the issue at hand.
   Can he or she tell you the basic facts of the situation?
   Can he or she describe what his or her choices are?
   Does he or she appreciate the ability to make choice and the risks and benefits of each choice? Does he or she know the consequences of not making a choice?
   Can he or she describe his or her reasoning in an organized, appropriate, and consistent manner?
   Is he or she able to express a choice?
4. Administer a cognitive screening test, such as the Mini-Mental State Examination.
5. Conduct a brief functional assessment relative to the issue at hand (e.g., for financial issues, ask the patient to describe how he or she accesses and manipulates his or her assets).
6. Make a determination of the patient's capacity to make decisions in an autonomous and reasonable manner relevant to the specific domains involved.

---

including *guardian, conservator,* and *fiduciary.* Surrogate decision makers can also be designated by individuals themselves before they become incapacitated. Typically, individuals use the form of a *durable power of attorney* to designate a family member to handle health care decisions or financial matters. The section on advance directives discusses health care surrogates in more detail.

CLINICAL VIGNETTE

Mr. Nicholas, a 78-year-old man, was involved in a motor vehicle accident in which he ran a stoplight and hit another car, injuring three people. He acted erratically afterward, sitting down on the ground when police tried to question him. He was arrested, but he managed to contact a friend to bail him out. A home visit by his attorney revealed a cluttered, unkempt house that was a clear fire hazard. Mr. Nicholas insisted on remaining in his home and resuming driving. His attorney wondered whether Mr. Nicholas could live alone anymore, drive, or even stand trial. When he was brought before the judge for an initial hearing, a psychiatric evaluation was ordered.

Dr. Stewart, the psychiatrist appointed by the court, interviewed Mr. Nicholas, his primary care physician, and a distant cousin. During the interview, Mr. Nicholas demonstrated poor short-term memory, and his factual account of the car accident was vague at best. He was unable to summarize what happened afterward, and he did not appreciate the severity of the charges against him. He reported that he was able to live alone, and he was oblivious to the poor condition of his house and his malnutrition. He scored 20 of a possible 30 points on the Mini-Mental State Examination. When Dr. Stewart asked Mr. Nicholas what would happen if he were to be convicted, he was unable to make a rational connection between the facts of the case and the potential legal consequences. Based on the forensic report, the judge declared Mr. Nicholas incompetent to stand trial and ordered that a guardian be appointed. He also mandated further evaluation in a geriatric psychiatry hospital unit. After a 4-week stay in which a diagnosis of probable Alzheimer disease (AD) was made, Mr. Nicholas's guardian moved him into a nursing home.

DIAGNOSTIC TRUTH TELLING

Families do not always want loved ones to know that they have dementia, especially AD, because of its prognosis. They may also choose not to tell the individual with dementia about a diagnosis of a terminal illness or a family crisis or tragedy. Some of the reasons to withhold such information are a desire to protect the individual from severe emotional reactions, as well as the belief that nothing can be gained by imparting information that the individual does not fully understand.

CLINICAL VIGNETTE

Mr. Emmett was an 83-year old man who lived with his wife in an assisted-living facility. Dr. Riles, his physician at the local Veterans Affairs hospital, expressed concern to Mr. Emmett and his wife about Mr. Emmett's memory, which seemed impaired. Dr. Riles later got a call from Mr. Emmett's son and daughter asking him not to tell Mr. Emmett or his wife that he may have something like AD, saying "they are happy now and enjoying their last years together—don't spoil it."

CLINICAL VIGNETTE

Mrs. Harrah was a 92-year-old woman with moderate to severe dementia. Her only daughter passed away, but her family members asked the staff not to inform her because the event might be too upsetting for her, if she even understood it at all. Nursing staff later reported that every few weeks Mrs. Harrah would ask when her daughter was coming to visit.

Whether to provide or withhold information in these cases and others depends on the degree of dementia, especially with respect to the individual's short-term memory and insight. Because individuals in early-stage dementia retain some degree of memory and insight into the diagnosis, most clinicians and dementia organizations recommend being truthful about a diagnosis, and they suggest that information on the nature of the disease, its prognosis, and the available treatments and support should be provided. Similarly, most clinicians encourage family members to tell individuals with early-stage dementia about important family crises or tragedies. Being truthful has numerous advantages, including the following.

- It may relieve the individual's anxiety and confusion over his or her symptoms of dementia or over the emotional reactions that he or she sees in other loved ones.
- It allows an individual to make important decisions about health care, estate planning, and life plans *before* they lose the capacity to do so.
- It affords the person the opportunity to make decisions about treatment options, including support groups and research studies.
- It enables the person to grieve the loss of a loved one or to provide support to those in crisis or grief.

As an individual's dementia increases, all of these advantages recede. The clinician then must make a judgment call about what is appropriate to tell the patient, including how much he or she needs to know.

IMPARTING BAD NEWS

Imparting information about a dementia diagnosis, a terminal disease, or a family crisis or tragedy must be done in a sensitive, humane, and thoughtful manner. The clinician should know ahead of time the individual's relative cognitive abilities so that he or she can make a judgment call about how much the individual can understand and at what level of detail. The clinician should never assume that, even in the advanced stages of dementia, the individual will not have an emotional reaction. Supportive family, friends, and staff should be present or immediately available. If the clinician anticipates a traumatic reaction from the individual, such as that which may occur in an individual with a history of depression or suicidality or when the loss is quite severe (e.g., the loss of an only child who was a primary support), he or she should have a mental health clinician available for consultation within hours. The clinician must also choose an appropriate time and location to meet so that privacy; confidentiality; and adequate time to relate the information, process it, and deal with the repercussions are ensured. Such information should never be provided over the phone, in a hallway, at the end of the day or work week, or without supports present. The necessary details should be given without any excessive elaboration that the patient will neither understand nor request; instead, the clinician should be prepared to provide additional details in response to questions that the individual may ask.

If the information is not imparted to the individual with dementia, he or she is potentially robbed of his or her autonomy to participate in personal and family decisions, as well as his or her right to prepare for death or to grieve a loss. Even in the advanced stages of dementia, an individual may retain the capacity to react to news and to grieve, although clinicians and family members may question whether any inherent good exists in putting someone through such pain if he or she does not truly understand nor retain the information.

GENETIC TESTING FOR ALZHEIMER DISEASE

At present, no genetic test or biomarker exists that can absolutely predict whether an individual will get AD (see Chapter 6 for more information). For most younger individuals, the only factors that may increase their risk of getting late-onset AD are family history and the presence of the APOE4 allele. However, an increased risk does not mean that someone will develop AD, and even knowing that one is homozygous for the APOE4 allele does not help in any way because no clear preventive strategy exists. If anything, the knowledge of increased risk may lead to excessive worry and overreactions to benign memory lapses. Moreover, such information in the wrong hands could ostensibly lead to discrimination or the denial of insurance. The only exception is individuals in particular family groupings with known genetic mutations for early-onset AD. However, individuals in those families usually know of their increased risk, and genetic testing is not always 100% accurate.

If an individual still requests genetic testing, he or she should have both pretest and posttest genetic counseling to aid in processing the results. At present, however, most individuals do not opt for testing, and the Alzheimer's Association and most clinicians do not recommend it. Of course, this situation will change when more accurate diagnostic testing and a way either to prevent or to treat AD definitively are available.

USE OF RESTRAINTS

Physical restraints were once commonly used in most nursing homes to keep agitated individuals from falling out of chairs or beds, pulling out tubes, or assaulting others. Types of physical restraints include vests with cords that are tied to a chair or bed, soft wrist restraints, and chairs with lap barriers. Over time, however, clinicians and researchers have recognized that restraints do not always decrease the occurrence of falls, injury, or agitation and that they can actually lead to increased injury and the overuse of psychotropic medications. In addition, restraints can be overly upsetting, frightening, and punitive for individuals, and they can result in excessive immobility, loss of function, and overdependency on staff. Great concern was also expressed over individuals who were being both physically and chemically restrained without adequate assessment and supervision. Consequently, most long-term care facilities are now restraint free. The only circumstances in which something like a soft lap restraint, which provides a barrier attached to a chair and not to the patient, may be appropriate are for those individuals who impulsively and repetitively make movements that would eject them from a wheelchair. The risk of injury in such a situation may be so great as to justify the use of a barrier; however, the patient must be under close supervision.

The use of psychotropic medications as chemical restraints raises similar issues, although the Omnibus Budget Reconciliation Act of 1987 guidelines provide appropriate restrictions (see Chapter 13). In general, the use of benzodiazepines and antipsychotic medications, especially in injectable forms, is discouraged, except in emergent situations; in these situations, they must be used with the knowledge and guidance of a psychiatrist or medically-trained clinician. Individuals who regularly require injectable medications should be more appropriately treated in inpatient psychiatric settings.

INFORMED CONSENT FOR TREATMENT AND RESEARCH

Informed consent is one of the foundations of the doctor–patient relationship. The responsibility of the clinician is to inform the patient of his or her condition and the risks and benefits of various treatment options as honestly and completely as possible and to obtain voluntary consent for treatment on that basis. Adequate information includes the name and characteristics of the diagnosis; its prognosis; the various treatment options, including their duration, risks, and benefits; and the consequences of no treatment. In addition, informed consent is frequently sought for patient participation in research studies looking at dementia and its associated conditions. For those individuals who have some capacity to understand their situation, regardless of whether they are making a treatment decision, discussing the diagnosis, treatment, and/or study protocol at their level of cognitive ability, without excessive detail that may confuse or frighten them, is important. This responsibility cannot always be discharged with patients with dementia, who may lack the capacity to understand, to appreciate, and to think rationally about their condition or treatment options. Instead, patients may refuse or may consent to treatment based on their physician's recommendations alone, their emotional reactions to how they understand the diagnosis, or distorted or delusional beliefs. In more severe states, they may lack the ability even to respond in a verbally coherent manner.

For all of these individuals, a surrogate is needed to aid them in making a decision. Ideally, the potential subject would have a living will that contains both treatment and research directives and that designates a surrogate. However, at this time, encountering such an individual is rare. In most states, consent for research is preferably provided by a legal guardian or an individual with durable power of attorney for health care, but it can also be given by an undesignated surrogate, such as a spouse or child, followed by a sibling or a close friend who serves as next of kin. Informed consent on the part of the surrogate requires that he or she fully understands the reason for the study, its risks and benefits, and his or her ability to refuse or withdraw consent at any point without fear of the patient's being denied alternate treatment. Research studies should be carried out only under the auspices of an institutional review board that monitors its protocol and the use of human subjects.

CLINICAL VIGNETTE

Mr. Badger, an 88-year-old man with vascular dementia and agitation, failed several antipsychotic medication trials. His psychiatrist, Dr. Milo, wanted to enroll him in a clinical trial of a new antipsychotic medication that was not yet on the market. Dr. Milo contacted Mr. Badger's son regarding his father's diagnosis of severe dementia and associated agitation. He proposed screening Mr. Badger for a study that involved a 10-week trial of an experimental medication versus a placebo, with the option of using open-label medication if no improvement is seen after 6 weeks. He reviewed the protocol as it was detailed in the informed consent, including the potential risks and benefits, compensation for potential injury, alternate treatments, the maintenance of confidentiality, the voluntary nature of consent, and ways to contact the investigator and his staff. Mr. Badger's son agreed to sign the consent form to enroll his father. Dr. Milo then explained to Mr. Badger that he would be giving him a medication to help him feel calmer and that he would be visiting him every week. "Oh great," said Mr. Badger, "Come and see me often!"

Not every study is appropriate for every patient with dementia. In general, if the study involves a minimal risk of harm to subjects, regardless of whether it may benefit them specifically, all patients with dementia can ethically be considered, preferably with the involvement of a surrogate decision maker. When a risk of harm is present, however, the decision to enroll should weigh the potential benefit to the subject. Enrollment is obviously considered more preferable when such a benefit exists, but, when it is unclear, the enrollment should be restricted to those individuals who can either consent themselves or who have executed a research-specific advance directive.

The use of placebos in studies raises specific ethical questions because patients may continue to suffer throughout the study without the possibility of therapeutic benefit. In general, the use of placebos is discouraged when a standard of care already exists. For example, if an accepted treatment for depression associated with dementia exists, denying this to a patient and instead allowing him or her to languish on a placebo are not ethical. The difficulty lies in defining a standard of care. For example, although no antipsychotic medication has been approved by the United States Food and Drug Administration for treating agitation associated with dementia, several are commonly used on an "off-label" basis, and the literature supporting their efficacy is growing. One could therefore argue that a standard of care does exist; others would disagree, stating that placebo-controlled trials of antipsychotics in this context are necessary because the data are not sufficient and because no United States Food and Drug Administration approval establishing standard treatment exists.

DRIVING

As the population ages, the number of older drivers has increased significantly. Although older drivers tend to be safer divers, they also have more fatalities per mile than younger drivers, except for young men ages 16 to 19 years old. Given the declines in cognitive skills essential for safe driving, older drivers with dementia pose a particular hazard above and beyond that in those individuals with the normal age-related risk factors for motor vehicle accidents, including decreased hearing and vision; physical disease and disability; slowed reaction time; and the effects of multiple medications, especially sedative-hypnotics. Clinical predictors of impaired driving include declines in an individual's short-term memory and decreases in his or her Mini-Mental State Examination scores. Neuropsychologic deficits of particular importance include those in visuospatial processing and frontal lobe functions, as these allow individuals to identify and attend to the most important elements in their visual field.

⊕ KEY POINT

Signs of impaired driving in individuals with dementia include driving too slowly; difficulty in making turns, lane changes, or exits; failing to observe traffic signs and rules of the road; becoming lost in familiar areas; slowed reaction to objects, other vehicles, or pedestrians in the road; leaving the car running or the keys in the ignition after stopping; forgetting to turn on the headlights at night or to fill up the gas tank; and improper or poor parking.

Despite these risk factors, after an individual has been licensed to drive, retesting (aside from visual acuity testing) is not obligatory in most states. In addition, older individuals are typically reluctant to give up driving even when they are told to do so, although many do moderate their driving anyway by driving less frequently at night, on freeways, or on unfamiliar roads. Giving up driving voluntarily or under duress can be devastating for an older individual because it harms his or her self-worth, robs the individual of his or her independence, increases his or her dependence on others, and makes going places and running errands difficult.

A diagnosis of dementia does not automatically disqualify someone from driving, but it does strongly indicate the need for limits, supervision, and alternate means of transportation. Ultimately, the individual must stop driving. When a clinician is concerned about a patient's capacity to drive, he or she should ask the patient and a reliable informant about pattern of driving, including frequency, time of day, weather and road conditions, destinations, type and condition of vehicle, and passengers, and for a history of his or her traffic violations and accidents. At the very least, the clinician should always recommend some form of functional assessment, specifically an on-road test by a qualified representative of the state's Department of Motor Vehicles. Some states *require* physicians to report impaired drivers for retesting. The problem is that this provision requires the physician to break patient–doctor confidentiality, so that the patient may no longer trust the physician or return for follow-up. Even worse, the individual may no longer be honest about his or her limitations. Regardless, the goal of intervention is to ensure the safety of the patient and others since the consequences of not intervening when an individual has become an impaired driver could be catastrophic.

⊕ KEY POINT

The American Academy of Neurology recommends that drivers with early-stage dementia undergo on-road retesting and regular reassessment every 6 months at a minimum, given the likely progression of the disease. Individuals with moderate to severe dementia should not be driving at all, given their significant impairment in driving performance and the increases in accident rates.

Unfortunately, a sizable percentage of patients with dementia ignores clinician recommendations and continues to drive in all circumstances. Even more alarming is the fact that many of these individuals and their caregivers believe that they can continue to drive throughout the course of their disease. As a result, the clinician's recommendations for a driver evaluation or for the patient to stop driving altogether frequently cause conflicts among clinicians, caregivers, and patients. To deal with these, clinicians should arm themselves with as much supporting data as possible, and they should document their recommendations carefully for the sake of risk management. Impaired individuals should be reported to the state's Department of Motor Vehicles, especially when this is mandated by state law. In extreme cases, caregivers may need to be instructed to take away the individual's car keys. For individuals with mild impairment, the clinician should always consider compromises, such as restricting driving to daylight hours in good weather and road conditions and only on well-recognized, less congested roads. Clinicians and caregivers should also take an active role in arranging alternative transportation for the patient so as not to leave him or her stranded. If the individual continues to drive, they should not be allowed to transport anyone (especially children), except for a caregiver who is aware of potential limitations.

CLINICAL VIGNETTE

Mr. Marquette, a 90-year-old man with a several-year history of slowed gait and memory loss, drove his car to take his wife shopping or on errands several times a week. He was pulled over by police because he was going the wrong way down a one-way street. A review of his driving record indicated that he had previously been cited for going 40 miles per hour on a freeway and for running a stop sign. Mr. Marquette referred the ticket to his nephew, an attorney, and asked him to take care of it. The nephew had suspected dementia in his uncle for some time, so he insisted that, as a condition of helping out with the ticket, Mr. Marquette had to undergo a dementia evaluation. Testing revealed relatively severe cognitive impairment, so, based on this, the nephew took away Mr. Marquette's car keys. He arranged, however, for a driver to take Mr. and Mrs. Marquette on errands several times a week. The nominal fee that the nephew took on himself to pay the driver was worth the peace of mind he would have, he figured, with regard to his worries that his uncle would injure or kill himself, his wife, or someone else.

The same concerns about driving apply to many other potentially hazardous activities that an individual with dementia may engage in, including the possession and use of firearms, child care, some sports (e.g., biking, skiing), driving boats and other recreational vehicles, and using power tools and yard equipment. All of these activities may require limitations and supervision in the early stages of dementia and prohibition later in the course of the illness.

SEXUAL RELATIONSHIPS

Individuals with dementia have the right to engage in sexual relationships with a partner, assuming both individuals have the capacity to understand the nature of the relationship and to provide consent. This issue often arises in relationships when a spouse or partner questions the ability of the other partner to provide consent or, in a long-term care setting, when two individuals with dementia are engaging in sexual activity. The latter situation often creates considerable anxiety on units, especially if one or more of the individuals has a spouse. In such situations, a psychiatric or psychologic consultation can help to determine the individuals' relative capacity to provide consent. As was noted before, the individual may lack capacity in many other areas, but he or she may still be able to consent to sex. When concerns arise, the clinician should question the individual to determine whether he or she knows the sexual partner and understands the nature of the relationship, including its risks, and whether he or she is able to refuse unwanted intimacy. In addition, the individual's current sexual behaviors should be compared with his or her past behaviors and known personal values.

ADVANCE DIRECTIVES

Advance directives are legal documents that are prepared and signed by an individual to indicate how medical decisions should be made for him or her if and when he or she becomes mentally incapacitated. They must be executed when an individual is still competent to make decisions. Advance directives are not unique to patients with dementia, and, since the enactment of the Patient Self-Determination Act in 1990, health care organizations are mandated to provide all patients with information on them. Advances directives may consist of the following:

- A *proxy directive* that designates a surrogate to make decisions for an individual in case he or she develops mental incapacity. The surrogate can be designated as a *durable power of attorney for heath care* or a *health care proxy*. Spouses and adult children are the individuals most commonly designated to serve as proxies, followed by parents, siblings, and other relatives.
- A *living will* that specifies an individual's wishes with respect to health care decisions when he or she lacks the mental capacity to make them.

Some of the medical issues that may be discussed in a living will include the following:

- Statement of religious principles or personal philosophy to guide medical decisions;
- Use of cardiopulmonary resuscitation and artificial respiration in case of cardiopulmonary arrest;
- Use of intravenous hydration and feeding tubes if the individual is unable to eat or drink;
- Use of artificial life support in case of a coma or persistent vegetative state;
- Participation in research studies;
- Permissibility of organ or tissue donation and autopsy.

Ideally, all individuals should prepare a document that includes a living will and designates a proxy to make health care decisions based on its guidelines. Without a living will, a designated proxy may make decisions inconsistent with the wishes of the patient; without a designated proxy, a living will must be interpreted by the next of kin who may or may not choose to honor its guidelines.

When an individual has no advance directives and he or she either has no next of kin or the family is unsure of what to do, medical decisions for the individual may be made based on his or her known values or religious beliefs, previous statements made with respect to end-of-life care, or ultimately what appears to be the most reasonable approach.

CLINICAL VIGNETTE

Mrs. Eugene, a 75-year-old woman with mild memory loss, had told her daughter that she was afraid of being kept alive "like a vegetable" and that she would like her to prevent unnecessary interventions when she could no longer make decisions. She did not want her son to make decisions for her because he had recently sustained a head injury and she did not trust his judgment. The son, however, told his sister that he was the oldest child and that he therefore had the right to make decisions for his mother. Mrs. Eugene signed a living will that specified her desire not to be put on artificial life support if she were in a terminal state. She also designated her daughter as her durable power of attorney for health care decisions.

CLINICAL VIGNETTE

Mr. Stone was an 85-year-old retired man with end-stage dementia. His swallowing ability had deteriorated, and he began refusing to eat. Before developing dementia, he had asked his physician never to put him on life support or artificial nutrition. However, he never wrote down his wishes or designated someone to decide in the event that he was incapacitated. His son insisted that a feeding tube be placed to keep him alive. Based on his son's wishes, Mr. Stone had a feeding tube placed. Even though his physician believed that Mr. Stone would have disagreed with this decision, he did not have any written statement to this effect, and he was obligated to honor the wishes of the son who was the next of kin.

END-OF-LIFE CARE

Despite their long courses, AD and other progressive dementias are terminal illnesses. In the last 6 to 12 months of life, patients with AD steadily enter a vegetative state as they lose their ability to communicate, to ambulate, and to swallow. Death often results from infection and malnutrition. However, medical technology has advanced considerably in the past few decades, and various interventions can now prolong this end stage for months. Although clinicians and caregivers seek to prevent pain and suffering during this stage, many question the value of prolonging the dying process when the individual has little perceived quality of life. Other individuals believe that the sanctity of life is paramount and that all efforts to prolong life should be exerted.

Advance directives play a key role in these situations, and all long-term care institutions request that families make decisions about *do not resuscitate*, or DNR, orders in the setting of end-stage dementia because the chances of recovery from cardiopulmonary arrest are slim. Caregivers need to understand, however, that DNR orders only apply to the use of cardiopulmonary resuscitation in emergent situations and that the use of other medical interventions can still be provided. For example, for physicians to discuss with caregivers how aggressively to treat superimposed medical conditions, such as infections, injuries (e.g., hip fracture), and malignancies, is important. The most common approach in end-stage dementia is to provide definitive treatment for minor problems that may otherwise cause undue pain or discomfort, such as coughs, small wounds or lacerations, constipation, diarrhea, and skin eruptions, and for more serious acute problems that cause significant suffering but that can be relieved with straightforward treatment, such as using a diuretic for pulmonary edema or a nebulizer treatment for an asthma attack. With more serious problems that require invasive treatment or surgery, such as fractures, malignancies, pneumonia, and myocardial infarction, the treatment approach is more often palliative, meaning that its aim is to relieve pain and to provide comfort without curing the problem. The issue becomes more controversial with an acute infection, such as pneumonia, that can be cured with a moderate degree of intervention but that otherwise may result in death within days. Even with advance directives, the emotional reactions to such situations can complicate decision making.

A similar ethical issue arises when an individual with dementia has dysphagia, making him or her at risk of choking and developing aspiration pneumonia. In the past, oral feeding was attempted as long as possible and was sometimes temporarily supplemented with nasogastric or intravenous nutrition. Since the 1980s, however, the placement of permanent feeding tubes directly through the abdominal wall and into the stomach has become more commonplace because of the development of percutaneous endoscopic gastrostomy, or PEG, tubes. These tubes allow indefinite nutritional supplementation. For many individuals without end-stage dementia, tube feeding can prolong life and can even provide a bridge of survival during recovery from a stroke or another illness that makes eating impossible.

For individuals with end-stage dementia, however, the survival benefit is less clear. The idea of not feeding someone and thus allowing him or her to die makes many clinicians and caregivers quite uncomfortable. Research suggests, however, that tube feeding in end-stage dementia does not necessarily enhance the individual's quality of life nor prolong his or her survival. In fact, it can be associated with uncomfortable symptoms, such as abdominal distention and cramping, aspiration, pain and infections at the tube site, nausea and vomiting, diarrhea, and agitation. Without artificial hydration and nutrition from tube feeding, death usually results within days. Although starvation is imagined to be painful, this is not necessarily true, perhaps in part because of the production of natural endorphins and the availability of supplemental morphine. Increasingly, hospice care has been playing a role in end-stage dementia, with the recognition that the goals of most families are palliation of pain and suffering and optimal comfort during the final days of life.

CLINICAL VIGNETTE

Mr. Bleyer, a 90-year-old man with moderate to severe dementia, was noted to be severely anemic. A stool guaiac was grossly positive, and subsequent abdominal computed tomography revealed a likely malignancy in his colon. In addition, Mr. Bleyer had contracted two bouts of pneumonia in the past year. His cognition had deteriorated greatly in the past 6 months, and, although he could still converse with the staff at his nursing home, the content of his speech was confused and disorganized. His physician, Dr. Green, requested a family meeting to discuss possible treatment for the cancer. The family met with Dr. Green, who presented the option of surgery with follow-up chemotherapy. The family did not want to put Mr. Bleyer through that, and it instead requested that he be kept comfortable with adequate pain control and hospice care. They agreed to a DNR order and requested that no medications or intravenous hydration be given in case of recurrent pneumonia. They based their decision on a living will that Mr. Bleyer had signed when he had been hospitalized several years before.

A GUIDE TO LEGAL PROTECTION

Based on the information in this chapter, all individuals should consider executing several of the following precautionary legal steps before the potential onset of dementia or, at the latest, during the early stages of disease with the assistance of a caregiver:

1. **Advance directives.** An individual should prepare a living will and should designate a durable power of attorney for health care decisions and research. He or she should specify that the power of attorney should follow the guidelines of the living will.
2. **Financial and estate planning.** The individual should prepare a will and should consider including a statement of capacity (with a videotape) if he or she is in the early stages of dementia. He or she should set up joint bank accounts with a spouse or a designated individual who then serves as a surrogate for the management of financial assets, and the individual should arrange for the direct deposit of pensions and other sources of income. He or she should designate a representative payee, if necessary, to manage his or her government benefits. These steps may prevent exploitation.
3. The individual should review his or her wishes with family members and designated proxies so that they understand his or her philosophy and can express any reservations about discharging them. If an individual distrusts a particular person, he or she should take the steps necessary to limit his or her involvement in decision making.

With advance directives and estate planning, an individual should consider consulting with competent, professional individuals with expertise in these areas. The Alzheimer's Association is a good first stop. For legal issues, the National Academy of Elder Law Attorneys can provide information and referrals by telephone (520-881-4005) or through their website (http://www.naela.com/). The website for Partnership in Caring: America's Voices for the Dying (http://www.part-nershipforcaring.org/) or their hotline (800-989-9455) can provide more information on advance directives.

The three steps listed are rapidly becoming standard for all adults, especially because health care institutions now provide information on advance directives every time someone is hospitalized. It is important for individuals to keep in mind that decision making during times of crisis or at the end of life may be influenced by strong emotions, family disputes, and situations that were not previously anticipated. Advance directives that include a living will and a designation of proxies can steer caregivers through these rough straits, but they must be coupled with open and honest communication between family and clinicians and an appeal to personal values and ethics that encompass the particulars of the situation.

APPENDICES

Pocket Cards:
Dementia Workup

CARD A.1. DEMENTIA SCREEN QUESTIONS

Check all that are present:

_____ Frequent forgetfulness that interferes with daily functioning
_____ Episodes of confusion to time and place
_____ Difficulty performing everyday tasks
_____ Difficulty remembering or choosing the right word
_____ Impaired recognition of familiar people or objects
_____ Episodes of poor or uncharacteristic decision making
_____ Impaired abstract thinking that interferes with complex tasks
_____ Agitated or inappropriate moods or behaviors

If you have checked one or more of these items, a dementia workup should be considered.

CARD A.2. THE DEMENTIA WORKUP: HISTORY

Introduction

- Build a rapport with the patient and informant and orient the patient to the interview.

History of Impairment

- Describe the cognitive impairment and the associated problems.
- When did it begin? Under what circumstances? How has it progressed?
- Describe the specific impairment in memory, orientation, language, recognition, motor tasks, judgment, abstract thinking, mood, behavior, and personality.
- Review relevant medical and psychiatric history and current medications.
- Review of systems: investigate all current physical and psychologic complaints.

Assessment of the Home Environment

- Is the individual engaging in risky behaviors?
- Is the home environment physically safe?
- Are signs of abuse, neglect, or exploitation observed?
- What are the mental and physical states of the caregiver?

CARD A.3. THE DEMENTIA WORKUP: PHYSICAL EXAMINATION

Physical Examination

1. Physical appearance
2. Vital signs
3. Head and neck
4. Lungs
5. Abdomen
6. Heart and pulses
7. Skin
8. Extremities and joints

Neurologic Examination

1. Cranial nerves I through XII
2. Motor system: strength, tone, atrophy, fasciculations, rigidity
3. Reflexes: biceps, triceps, knee, ankle, Babinski
4. Sensory system: touch, pain and/or temperature, vibratory, positional, Romberg
5. Cerebellar system: ataxia, dysmetria, intention tremor, dysarthria, nystagmus
6. Gait: parkinsonian, ataxic, unsteady, cerebellar, spastic
7. Abnormal movements: dyskinesia, dystonia, tremor, bradykinesia, chorea, myoclonus
8. Frontal release signs: glabellar, snout, palmomental, suck, root, grasp, perseveration

CARD A.4. THE DEMENTIA WORKUP: MENTAL STATUS EXAMINATION

Mental Status Examination

1. Appearance: normal, disheveled, disorganized, malodorous
2. Behavior and attitude: cooperative, apathetic, resistant, agitated
3. Speech: coherent, dysarthric, pressured, echolalia, mute
4. Language: normal, aphasic
5. Affect and mood: neutral, depressed, anxious, irritable, blunted, flat
6. Thought process: coherent, disorganized, flight of ideas, tangential
7. Thought content: obsessions, delusions (paranoid, grandiose, bizarre), hallucinations, suicidality, homicidality
8. Cognitive screen: orientation, attention, concentration, memory, abstraction, insight, judgment; Mini-Mental State Examination; Clock Drawing Test (Card A.4a)

CARD A.4A. THE COGNITIVE SCREEN FOR DEMENTIA

Step 1

Administer a brief cognitive screening instrument. Examples include the Mini-Mental State Examination (30-point scale), the Mini-Cog (rates patient as *probably demented* or *probably not demented*), and/or the Clock Drawing Test (provides a general impression; can be scored; see Card A.4B).

Step 2

Look for evidence of the following diagnostic hallmarks of dementia in the mental status examination and on the screening instrument:

Memory impairment

- Poor 3-item repetition and recall
- Poor recall of important recent and remote events

Language Impairment (Aphasia)

- Difficulty understanding and repeating words or instructions (e.g., incorrect or no response to requests, responses consisting of unintelligible or jumbled words or phrases, minimal verbal responses)
- Difficulty generating lists of words

Impaired Motor Ability (Apraxia)

- Poor ability to copy a design or to draw a clock face
- Difficulty imitating or demonstrating movements (e.g., hand movements, combing hair, brushing teeth)

Impaired Recognition (Agnosia)

- Impaired orientation in familiar surroundings
- Impaired recognition of familiar objects or people

Executive Dysfunction

- Difficulty with tasks that require organization (e.g., drawing time on clock, managing medications or household chores, balancing checkbook)
- Repetitive or perseverated language or behaviors

CARD A.4B. CLOCK DRAWING TEST

Instructions

Draw the face of a clock with the numbers on it. Then, draw the hands on the clock so that the time reads as 11:10.

Scoring Method 1 : 4-Point Scale

Score one point for the correct representation of the following four factors: (a) the clock face drawn as circle, (b) the numbers in the correct positions, (c) all 12 numbers included, and (d) hands in the correct position.

Scoring Method 2: 10-Point Scale*

Clock face: Score 0 to 2 based on degree of distortion (0, absent or totally distorted; 1, incomplete, some distortion; 2, intact).

Numbers on the clock: Score 0 to 4 based on proper number list, sequencing, and placement (0, absent or hardly placed; 1, missing or added numbers, major distortions; 2, missing or added numbers, spatial distortions; 3, numbers present but spatial distortions; 4, numbers all present and spatially correct).

Hands of the clock: Score 0 to 4 based on presence and placement (0, no hands or grossly distorted representations; 1, only one hand or grossly distorted two hands; 2, both hands present but placed incorrectly; 3, mild errors in placement or unable to differentiate minute from hour hand; 4, correct placement and size difference in hand).

Interpretation: A score of 9 to 10 is considered normal; scores less than 7 demonstrate mild to severe impairment.

---

*From Rouleau I, Salmon DP, Butters N, et al. Quantitative and qualitative analyses of clock drawings in Alzheimer's disease and Huntington's disease. *Brain Cogn* 1992;18:70–87, with permission.

CARD A.5. THE DEMENTIA WORKUP: TESTS

Laboratory Tests

Complete blood count, electrolytes, glucose, blood urea nitrogen (BUN) and creatinine, calcium, thyroid-stimulating hormone (TSH), liver function tests (LFTs), erythrocyte sedimentation rate (ESR), vitamin B_{12}, folate, rapid plasmin reagin (RPR), urinalysis (UA)

Toxicology screen and heavy metal screen, if suspected

Lumbar puncture if encephalitis is suspected

Brain Computed Tomography or Magnetic Resonance Imaging

Computed tomography without contrast for routine screen

Magnetic resonance imaging to focus on white matter lesions, small infarcts, and lesions in brainstem or subcortical regions

Electroencephalography

To look for focal lesions and seizure activity and to differentiate dementia from delirium

Neuropsychologic Testing

General cognitive screen: Mini-Mental State Examination, Clock Drawing Test

Selected tests per the neuropsychologist

Functional Testing

Selected by the neuropsychologist

Pocket Cards:
Agitation, Psychosis, and
Delirium in Dementia

CARD B.1. ASSESSMENT OF AGITATION AND PSYCHOSIS IN DEMENTIA

Use the ABCs mnemonic for assessment.

Antecedents

- What factors preceded or appeared to trigger disturbances?

Behaviors

- Describe the disturbances based on observations and reports.

Concurrent or Comorbid Stresses

- Look for concurrent environmental stresses or comorbid medical or psychiatric disorders.

Consequences

- What results from the behaviors? Is someone being harmed? Are they reinforced in any way?

Major Causes of Agitation and Psychosis

Major causes include the following:

(a) dementia itself
(b) medical illness
(c) delirium
(d) medications
(e) pain
(f) psychiatric illness
(g) sleep problems, and
(h) stress.

CARD B.2. CONFUSION ASSESSMENT METHOD RATING SCALE FOR DELIRIUM*

Instruments: Consider a diagnosis of delirium if features 1 and 2 and either feature 3 or 4 are present:

Feature 1: Acute Onset and Fluctuating Course

Look for evidence of an acute change in mental status from baseline, with fluctuations in associated abnormal behaviors.

Feature 2: Inattention

Observe the patient for difficulty in focusing attention or keeping track of conversations.

Feature 3: Disorganized Thinking

Look for disorganized or incoherent thinking, rambling conversation, illogical flow of ideas, or unpredictable switching from subject to subject.

Feature 4: Altered Level of Consciousness

Is the level of consciousness anything other than alert? Examples are vigilant, lethargic, stuporous, and comatose.

---

*Based on Inouye SK, van Dyck CH, Alessi CA, et al. Clarifying confusion: the confusion assessment method: a new method for detection of delirium. *Ann Intern Med* 1990;113:941–948.

CARD B.3. TREATMENT OF AGITATION AND PSYCHOSIS IN DEMENTIA

Treatment should be based on the mnemonic TREAT:

Target: define target symptoms.
Reversible causes: treat reversible causes.
Environment: optimize the environment; consider a behavioral plan.
Agents: select an appropriate psychopharmacologic agent.
Try again: if improvement is insufficient, try again.

Strategies for Treatment-Resistant Symptoms

- Reassess for untreated medical or psychiatric problems and persistent environmental triggers;
- Refocus the environmental or behavioral plan;
- Reassess the medication trial for adequate dose and duration, proper dispensing, compliance, and paradoxical side effects;
- Consider the use of an alternate medication or augmentation of existing agent.

Behavioral Crises

For behavioral crises, follow the mnemonic CALM:

Calm the individual with a gentle approach;
Assess the environment for immediate triggers;
Limit access to unsafe places or situations;
Medicate as necessary.

CARD B.4. OBRA, OR OMNIBUS BUDGET RECONCILIATION ACT OF 1987, GUIDELINES*

The following documentation is required for a long-term care resident on anxiolytic, sedative/hypnotic, and antipsychotic medications:

Diagnostic Indications for Antipsychotic Medications

1. Psychotic disorders (schizophrenia and others in the *Diagnostic and Statistical Manual of Mental Disorders*, Fourth Edition, Text Revision)
2. Organic mental syndromes (dementia or delirium associated with agitation or psychosis)
3. Other: Huntington disease; Tourette syndrome; or short-term treatment of hiccups, nausea, vomiting, or pruritus

Diagnostic Indications for Anxiolytics or Sedative-Hypnotics:

1. Generalized anxiety disorder
2. Panic disorder
3. Organic mental syndromes (as above)
4. Symptomatic anxiety associated with other psychiatric disorders
5. Short-term treatment of insomnia (10 days)

Target Symptoms

Note if they are better, worse, or unchanged.

Behavioral Interventions

Document nonpharmacologic attempts to treat behavioral symptoms.

Medications

1. Note name, dose, and side effects (extrapyramidal symptoms and tardive dyskinesia for antipsychotics)
2. Attempt to taper each medication after the initial 4 months and then at least twice per year
3. Include rationale for doses that are above suggested limits

---

*Based on Omnibus Budget Reconciliation Act of 1987: subtitle C, nursing home reform: PL100-203. Washington, D.C.: National Coalition for Nursing Home Reform, 1987.

CARD B.5 OBRA, OR OMNIBUS BUDGET RECONCILIATION ACT OF 1987, DOSING GUIDELINES

Drug	Maximum dose (mg per day)*
Short-acting benzodiazepines	
Lorazepam (Ativan)	2 (1)
Oxazepam (Serax)	30 (15)
Alprazolam (Xanax)	0.75 (0.25)
Long-acting Benzodiazepines	
Clonazepam (Klonopin)	1.5
Chlordiazepoxide (Librium)	20
Clorazepate (Tranxene)	15
Diazepam (Valium)	5
Hypnotics	
Triazolam (Halcion)	0.125
Temazepam (Restoril)	15
Flurazepam (Dalmane)	15
Anxiolytics and sedatives	
Hydroxyzine (Atarax , Vistaril)	50 (50)
Diphenhydramine (Benadryl)	50 (25)
Buspirone (Buspar)	30
Chloral hydrate	750 (500)
Conventional antipsychotics	
Haloperidol (Haldol)	4
Fluphenazine (Prolixin)	4
Thiothixene (Navane)	7
Perphenazine (Trilafon)	8
Trifluoperazine (Stelazine)	8
Thioridazine (Mellaril)	75
Chlorpromazine (Thorazine)	75
Atypical antipsychotics	
Clozapine (Clozaril)	50
Risperidone (Risperdal)	2
Olanzapine (Zyprexa)	10
Quetiapine (Seroquel)	200

*Doses in parentheses represent maximal doses for hypnotic use

Pocket Cards:
Depression in Dementia

CARD C.1. ASSESSMENT OF DEPRESSION IN DEMENTIA

1. Obtain clinical history and mental status examination.
2. Review depression symptom checklist (Card C.2).
3. Look for common dementia-related symptoms of depression.

   Affect and mood: sadness or uncharacteristic irritability, unreasonableness, or passivity

   Response style: poor attempts to provide answers

   Thought content: preoccupation with somatic symptoms or pain; excessive thoughts and comments about deceased relatives, personal losses, or death; and somatic delusions

   Behaviors: agitation, isolative behaviors, noncompliance, slow progress in rehabilitation, failure to thrive, indirect life-threatening behaviors

4. Review differential diagnosis to determine whether dementia alone, dementia with depression, pseudodementia (depression-induced cognitive impairment), apathy (impairment in motivation, not mood), or complicated bereavement is present.
5. Conduct physical and neurologic examination, routine laboratory tests, and other relevant tests.

CARD C.2. DEPRESSION SYMPTOM CHECKLIST FOR DEMENTIA

Check all that are present:

_____ Persistently sad or depressed mood
_____ Feelings of hopelessness and helplessness
_____ Decreased concentration
_____ Suicidal ideation
_____ Insomnia
_____ Decreased energy or activity level
_____ Psychomotor retardation
_____ Loss of interest in previously enjoyed activities
_____ Loss of pleasure in previously enjoyed activities
_____ Agitation and restlessness
_____ Anxiety or panic symptoms
_____ Multiple new somatic complaints
_____ Loss of appetite or weight loss
_____ Paranoid ideation

Suspect depression when the first item and one or more of the other items are checked.

CARD C.3. PSYCHOPHARMACOLOGIC TREATMENT OF DEPRESSION IN DEMENTIA

First-line agents: selective serotonin reuptake inhibitor (SSRI) or mirtazapine (Remeron) or venlafaxine (Effexor XR)

Second-line agents: venlafaxine or bupropion (Wellbutrin SR) or nefazodone (Serzone)

Third-line agents: psychostimulant (methylphenidate preferred) or tricyclic antidepressant; nortriptyline (Pamelor) or desipramine (Norpramin) preferred

Strategies for Treatment-Resistant Depression

1. Reassess to ensure adequate dose and length of trial, proper administration, and compliance.
2. Add a behavioral plan or some form of therapeutic contact.
3. Try a different antidepressant.
4. Augment the antidepressant: (a) SSRI plus mirtazapine, venlafaxine, or bupropion; (b) mirtazapine plus venlafaxine; (c) SSRI plus an atypical antipsychotic or a mood stabilizer.
5. Consider electroconvulsive therapy for intractable or life-threatening symptoms.

Pocket Card:
Caregiver Assessment

CARD D.1. THE MINI-BURDEN INTERVIEW

Perceptions and Experience of Burden

1. Do you feel you are under significant stress? If yes, describe.
2. Do you feel depressed? Anxious? To what degree?
3. Have you had difficulty sleeping? Eating?
4. Do you have more medical problems than before?
5. Do you constantly feel exhausted?
6. Have you felt that life is not worth living? Suicidal?
7. Have you ever felt like hitting or even ending the life of your loved one with dementia?

Potential Causes of Burden

8. Do you need more visitors ? More assistance? More time for yourself?
9. Does your loved one have behavioral problems? Paranoia?
10. Is he or she depressed? Apathetic?

The greater the number of yes responses is, the greater the likelihood of increased burden and the need for active intervention.

Suggested Readings

Alexopoulos GS, Silver JM, Kahn DA, et al. The expert consensus guideline series: treatment of agitation in older persons with dementia. *Postgrad Med* 1998;Spec No:1–88.

Campbell JJ, Duffy JD. Treatment strategies in amotivated patients. *Psychiatr Ann* 1997;27:44–49.

Cantor MD, Kayser-Jones J, Finucane TE. To force feed the patient with dementia or not to feed: preferences, evidence base, and regulation. *Ann Long Term Care* 2002;10:45–48.

Carlat DJ. *Practical guides in psychiatry: the psychiatric interview.* Baltimore: Lippincott Williams & Wilkins, 1999.

Cohen-Mansfield J. Nonpharmacologic interventions for inappropriate behaviors in dementia: a review, summary, and critique. *Am J Geriatr Psychiatry* 2001;9:361–381.

Cummings JL. Cholinesterase inhibitors: a new class of psychotropic compounds. *Am J Psychiatry* 2000;157:4–15.

Dunkin JJ, Anderson-Hanley C. Dementia caregiver burden: a review of the literature and guidelines for assessment and intervention. *Neurology* 1998;51:S53–S60.

Fields RB, Cisewski D, Coffey CE. Traumatic brain injury. In: Coffey EC, Cummings JL, eds. *Textbook of geriatric neuropsychiatry,* 2nd ed. Washington, D.C.: American Psychiatric Press, 2000:621–654.

Fisher JW. Legal aspects of the psychosocial management of the demented patient. *Psychiatr Ann* 1994;24:197–201.

Informed consent for research on human subjects with dementia. AGS Ethics Committee. American Geriatrics Society. *J Am Geriatr Soc* 1998;46:1308–1310.

Katz IR. Diagnosis and treatment of depression in patients with Alzheimer's disease and other dementias. *J Clin Psychiatry* 1998;59:38–44.

Kertesz A, Martinez-Lange P, Davidson W, et al. The corticobasal degeneration syndrome overlaps progressive aphasia and frontotemporal dementia. *Neurology* 2000;55:1368–1375.

Kertesz A, Munoz DG. Frontotemporal dementia. *Med Clin North Am* 2002;86:501–518.

Knopman DS. Alzheimer's disease and dementia: an overview of common non-Alzheimer dementias. *Clin Geriatr Med* 2001;17:281–301.

Mace NL, Rabins PV. *The 36-hour day: a family guide to caring for persons with Alzheimer's disease, related dementing illness, and memory loss in later life,* revised edition. Baltimore: John Hopkins University Press, 1999.

Malloy PF, Cohen RA, Jenkins MA. Frontal lobe function and dysfunction. In: Snyder PJ, Nussbaum PD, eds. *Clinical neuropsychol-*

ogy: a pocket handbook for assessment. Washington, D.C.: American Psychological Association, 1998:573–590.

McKeith IG, Burn D. Spectrum of Parkinson's disease, Parkinson's dementia, and Lewy body dementia. *Neurol Clin* 2000;18:865–902.

McKeith IG, Galasko D, Kosaka K, et al. Consensus guidelines for the clinical and pathologic diagnosis of dementia with Lewy bodies (DLB): report of the consortium on DLB international workshop. *Neurology* 1996;47:1113–1124.

McKeith IG, Perry EK, Perry RH. Report of the second dementia with Lewy body international workshop: diagnosis and treatment. Consortium on Dementia and Lewy Bodies. *Neurology* 1999;53: 902–905.

McKhann GM, Albert MS, Grossman M, et al. Clinical and pathological diagnosis of frontotemporal dementia: report of the Work Group on Frontotemporal Dementia and Pick's Disease. *Arch Neurol* 2001;58:1803–1809.

Mittelman MS, Epstein C, Pierzchala A. *Counseling the Alzheimer's caregiver: a resource for healthcare professionals*. Chicago, IL: American Medical Association Press, 2002.

Post SG. Key issues in the ethics of dementia care. *Neurol Clin* 2000; 18:1011–1022.

Roman GC. Vascular dementia revisited: diagnosis, pathogenesis, treatment, and prevention. *Med Clin North Am* 2002;86:477–499.

Roman GC, Tatemichi TK, Erkinjuntti T, et al. Vascular dementia: diagnostic criteria for research studies. Report of the NINDS-AIREN International Workshop. *Neurology* 1993;43:250–260.

Ross GW, Bowen JD. The diagnosis and differential diagnosis of dementia. *Med Clin North Am* 2002;86:455–476.

Scharre DW. Neoplastic, demyelinating, infectious, and inflammatory brain disorders. In: Coffey CE, Cummings JL, eds. *Textbook of geriatric neuropsychiatry*, 2nd ed. Washington, D.C.: American Psychiatric Press, 2000:669–697.

Schulz R, Beach SR. Caregiving as a risk factor for mortality. The Caregiver Health Effects Study. *JAMA* 1999;282:2215–2219.

Shenk D. *The forgetting. Alzheimer's: portrait of an epidemic*. New York: Doubleday, 2001.

Snowdon D. *Aging with grace. What the Nun Study teaches us about leading longer, healthier, and more meaningful lives*. New York: Bantam Books, 2001.

Snyder L. *Speaking our minds: personal reflections from individuals with Alzheimer's*. New York: WH Freeman, 2000.

Spar JE. Competency and related forensic issues. In: Coffey CE, Cummings JL, eds. *Textbook of geriatric neuropsychiatry*, 2nd ed. Washington, D.C.: American Psychiatric Press, 2000:945–963.

Tariot PN. Treatment of agitation in dementia. *J Clin Psychiatry* 1999; 60:11–20.

Trzepacz PT. Delirium. Advances in diagnosis, pathophysiology, and treatment. *Psychiatr Clin North Am* 1996;19: 429–448.

Whitehouse PJ. Ethical issues. In: Coffey CE, Cummings JL, eds. *Textbook of geriatric neuropsychiatry*, 2nd ed. Washington, D.C.: American Psychiatric Press, 2000:935–994.

Zgola JM, Mace NL. *Doing things: a guide to programming activities for persons with Alzheimer's disease and related disorders*. Baltimore: Johns Hopkins University Press, 1987.

Sources for Resource Materials Discussed in Text

Alexopoulos GS, Abrams RC, Young RC, Shamoian CA. Cornell Scale for Depression in Dementia. *Biol Psychiatry* 1988;23:271–284.

Allen CK, Allen RE. Cognitive disabilities: measuring the social consequences of mental disorders. *J Clin Psychiatry* 1987;48:185–190.

Berberger-Gateau P, Dartigues JF, Letenneur L. Four Instrumental Activities of Daily Living Score as a predictor of one-year incident dementia. *Age Ageing* 1993;22:457–463.

Blessed G, Tomlinson BE, Roth M. The association between quantitative measures of dementia and of senile change in the cerebral gray matter of elderly subjects. *Br J Psychiatry* 1968;114;797– 811.

Borson S, Scanlan J, Brush M, et al. The Mini-Cog: a cognitive 'vital signs' measure for dementia screening in multi-lingual elderly. *Int J Geriatr Psychiatry* 2000;15:1021–1027.

Burns T, Mortimer JA, Merchak P. Cognitive Performance Test: a new approach to functional assessment in Alzheimer's disease. *J Geriatr Psychiatry Neurol* 1994;7:46–54.

Cohen-Mansfield J. *Instruction manual for the Cohen-Mansfield Agitation Inventory (CMAI)*. Rockville, MD: The Research Institute of the Hebrew Home of Greater Washington, 1991

Cole M, Dastoor D. The Hierarchic Dementia Rating Scale. *J Clin Exper Gerontol* 1983;5:219–234.

Cummings JL, Mega M, Gray K, et al. The Neuropsychiatric Inventory: comprehensive assessment of psychopathology in dementia. *Neurology* 1994;44:2308–2314.

DeJong R, Osterlund O, Roy G. Measurement of quality-of-life changes in patients with Alzheimer's disease. *Clin Ther* 1989;11: 545–554.

Drachman DA, Swearer JM. Screening for dementia: Cognitive Assessment Screening Test (CAST). *Am Fam Physician* 1996;54: 1957–1964.

Dubois B, Slachevsky A, Litvan I, Pillon B. The FAB: a Frontal Assessment Battery at bedside. *Neurology* 2000;55:1621–1626.

Folstein MF, Folstein SE, McHugh PR. "Mini-Mental State": a practical method for grading the cognitive state of patients for the clinician. *J Psychiatr Res* 1975;12:189–198.

Froehlich TE, Robison JT, Inouye SK. Screening for dementia in the outpatient setting: the Time and Change test. *J Am Geriatr Soc* 1998;46:1506 – 1511.

Gelinas G, et al. Assessment of functional disability in Alzheimer's disease. *Can J Occup Ther* 1995;62(suppl):15.

Hachinski VC, Iliff LD, Zilhka E, et al. Cerebral blood flow in dementia. *Arch Neurol* 1975;32:632–637.

Hamilton M. A rating scale for depression. *J Neurol Neurosurg Psychiatry* 1960;23:56–62.

Inouye SK, van Dyck CH, Alessi CA, et al. Clarifying confusion: the confusion assessment method. A new method for detection of delirium. *Ann Intern Med* 1990;113:941–948.

Katzman R, Brown T, Fuld P, et al. Validation of a short orientation-memory-concentration test of cognitive impairment. *Am J Psychiatry* 1983;140:734–749.

Kiernan RJ, Mueller J, Langston JW, et al. The Neurobehavioral Cognitve Status Examination: a brief but differentiated approach to cognitive assessment. *Ann Intern Med* 1987;107:481–485.

Kokmen F, Naessens JM, Offord KP. A short test of mental status: description and preliminary results. *Mayo Clinic Proc* 1987;62:281–288.

Lawton MP, Brody EM. Assessment of older people: self-maintaining and instrumental activities of daily living. *Gerontologist* 1969;9:179–186.

Levin HS, High WM, Goethe KE, et al. The Neurobehavioral Rating Scale: assessment of the behavioral sequelae of head injury by the clinician. *J Neurol Neurosurg Psychiatry* 1987;50:183–193.

Mattis S. Mental status examination for organic mental syndrome in the elderly patient. In: Bellak R, Karasu TE, eds. *Geriatric psychiatry*. New York: Grune & Stratton, 1976:77–121.

McGivney SA, Mulvihill M, Taylor B. Validating the GDS depression screen in the nursing home. *J Am Geriatr Soc* 1994;42:490–492.

Morris JC. The Clinical Dementia Rating (CDR): current version and scoring rules. *Neurology* 1993;42:2412–2414.

Overall JE, Beller SA. The Brief Psychiatric Rating Scale (BPRS) in geropsychiatrics research: I. Factor structures on inpatient unit. *J Gerontol* 1984;39:187–193.

Overall JE, Gorham DR. The Brief Psychiatric Rating Scale. *Psychol Rep* 1962;10:799–812.

Patel V, Hope R. A rating scale for aggressive behaviour in the elderly—The RAGE. *Psych Med* 1992;22:211–221.

Pfeffer RI, Kurosaki TT, Harrah CH, et al. Measurement of functional activities in older adults in the community. *J Gerontol* 1982; 37:323–329.

Reisberg B. Functional assessment staging (FAST). *Psychopharmacol Bull* 1988;24:653–659.

Reisberg B, Auer SR, Monteiro M. Behavioral pathology in Alzheimer's disease (BEHAVE-AD) rating scale. *Int Psychogeriatr* 1996;3:301–308.

Reisberg B, Ferris SH, de Leon MJ, et al. The Global Deterioration Scale for assessment of primary degenerative dementia. *Am J Psychiatry* 1982;139:1136–1139.

Reisberg B, Schneck MK, Ferris SH, et al. The Brief Cognitive Rating Scale (BCRS): findings in primary degenerative dementia (PDD). *Psychopharmacol Bull* 1983;19:47–50.

Rosen WG, Mohs RC, Davis KL. A new rating scale for Alzheimer's disease. *Am J Psychiatry* 1984;141:1356–1364.

Royall DR, Mahurin RK, Gray KF. Bedside assessment of executive cognitive impairment: the executive interview. *J Am Geriatr Soc* 1992;40:1221–1226.

Solomon PR, Hirschoff A, Kelly B, et al. A 7-minute neurocognitive screening battery highly sensitive to Alzheimer's disease. *Arch Neurol* 1998;55:349–355.

Sultzer DL, Levin HS, Mahler ME, et al. Assessment of cognitive, psychiatric, and behavioral disturbances in patients with dementia: the Neurobehavioral Rating Scale. *J Am Geriatr Soc* 1992;40: 549–555.

Sunderland T, Alterman IS, Yount D, et al. A new scale for the assessment of depressed moods in demented patients. *Am J Psychiatry* 1988;145:955–959.

Tariot PN, Mack JL, Patterson MB, et al. The Behavior Rating Scale for Dementia of the Consortium to Establish a Registry for Alzheimer's Disease. The Behavior Pathology Committee of the Consortium to Establish a Registry for Alzheimer's Disease. *Am J Psychiatry* 1995;152:1349–1357.

Teng EL, Chui HC. The Modified Mini-Mental State (3MS) Examination. *J Clin Psychiatry* 1987;48:314–318.

Teunisse S, Derix MM, van Crevel H. Assessing the severity of dementia. Patient and caregiver. *Arch Neurol* 1991;48:274–277.

Trzepacz PT. The Delirium Rating Scale. Its use in consultation-liaison research. *Psychosomatics* 1999;40:193–204.

Trzepacz PT, Baker RW, Greenhouse J. A symptom rating scale for delirium. *Psychiatric Res* 1988;23:89–97.

Vitaliano PP, Russo J, Young HM, et al. The screen for caregiver burden. *Gerontologist* 1991;31:76–83.

Yesavage JA, Brink TL, Rose TL, et al. Development and validation of a geriatric depression screening scale: a preliminary report. *J Psychiatr Res* 1982-1983;17:37–49.

Yudofsky S, Silver J, Hales R. The Overt Aggression Scale for objective rating of verbal and physical aggression. *Am J Psychiatry* 1986;143:35–39.

Zarit SH, Reever KE, Bach-Peterson J. Relatives of the impaired elderly: correlates of feelings of burden. *Gerontologist* 1980;20:649–655.

Subject Index

Note: Page numbers followed by an *f* indicate figures; those followed by a *t* indicate tables